Navigating Life
with Migraine
and Other Headaches

Lisa M. Shulman, MD

Editor-in-Chief, *Neurology Now*™ Books Series
Fellow of the American Academy of Neurology
Professor of Neurology
The Eugenia Brin Professor in Parkinson's Disease and Movement Disorders
The Rosalyn Newman Distinguished Scholar in Parkinson's Disease
Director, University of Maryland Parkinson's Disease and Movement
Disorders Center
University of Maryland School of Medicine
Baltimore, MD

Other Titles in the *Neurology Now*™ Books Series

Navigating Life with Parkinson Disease
Sotirios A. Parashos, MD, PhD; Rose Wichmann, PT; and Todd Melby

Navigating Life with a Brain Tumor
Lynne P. Taylor, MD, FAAN; Alyx B. Porter Umphrey, MD; and Diane Richard

Navigating the Complexities of Stroke
Louis R. Caplan, MD, FAAN

Navigating Life with Multiple Sclerosis
Kathleen Costello, MS, ANP- BC, MSCN; Ben W. Thrower, MD;
and Barbara S. Giesser, MD

Navigating Life with Epilepsy
David C. Spencer, MD, FAAN

Navigating Life with Amyotrophic Lateral Sclerosis
Mark B. Bromberg, MD, PhD, FAAN, and Diane Banks Bromberg, JD

Navigating Life with Migraine and Other Headaches

William B. Young, MD, FAHS, FAAN

Professor of Neurology
Thomas Jefferson University
Jefferson Hospital for Neuroscience
Philadelphia, PA

Stephen D. Silberstein, MD, FAHS, FAAN, FACP

Professor of Neurology
Thomas Jefferson University
Jefferson Hospital for Neuroscience
Philadelphia, PA

AMERICAN ACADEMY OF
NEUROLOGY.

OXFORD
UNIVERSITY PRESS

Oxford University Press is a department of the University of Oxford. It furthers
the University's objective of excellence in research, scholarship, and education
by publishing worldwide. Oxford is a registered trade mark of Oxford University
Press in the UK and certain other countries.

Published in the United States of America by Oxford University Press
198 Madison Avenue, New York, NY 10016, United States of America.

Library of Congress Cataloging-in-Publication Data
Names: Young, William B. (William Boyd), 1959– author. |
Silberstein, Stephen D., author. | American Academy of Neurology, issuing body.
Title: Navigating life with migraine and other headaches / by William B. Young
and Stephen D. Silberstein.
Other titles: Neurology now books.
Description: [Minneapolis, Minn.] : American Academy of Neurology ;
New York, NY : Oxford University Press, [2018] |
Series: Neurology now books | Includes index.
Identifiers: LCCN 2017009335 | ISBN 9780190640767 (paperback : alk. paper)
Subjects: | MESH: Headache Disorders—therapy | Migraine Disorders—therapy |
Popular Works
Classification: LCC RC392 | NLM WL 342 | DDC 616.8/4912—dc23
LC record available at https://lccn.loc.gov/2017009335

1 3 5 7 9 8 6 4 2
Printed by Sheridan Books, Inc., United States of America

CONTENTS

ABOUT THE AAN'S *NEUROLOGY NOW*™ BOOKS SERIES

Here is a question for you:

If you know more about your neurologic condition, will you do better than if you know less?

Well, not simply optimism but hard data show that individuals who are more knowledgeable about their medical conditions do have better outcomes. So learning about your neurologic condition plays an important role in doing the very best you can. The main purpose of both the *Neurology Now*™ Books series and *Neurology Now* magazine from American Academy of Neurology (AAN) is to focus on the needs of people with neurologic disorders. Our goal is to view neurologic issues through the eyes of people with neurologic problems in order to understand and respond to their practical day-to-day needs.

So, you are probably saying, "Of course, knowledge is a good thing, but how can it change the course of my disease?" Well, health care is really a two-way street. After you have had a stroke, you need to find a knowledgeable and trusted neurologist; however, no physician can overcome the obstacle of working with inaccurate or incomplete information. Your physician is working to navigate the clues you provide in your own words combined with the clues from their neurologic examination in order to arrive at an accurate diagnosis and respond to your individual needs. Many types of important clues exist, such as your description of your symptoms or your ability to identify how your neurologic condition affects your daily activities.

Poor patient-physician communication inevitably results in less-than-ideal outcomes. This problem is well described by the old adage, "garbage in, garbage out." The better you pin down and communicate your main problem(s), the more likely you are to walk out of your doctor's office with the plan that is right for you. Your neurologist is the expert in your disorder, but you and your family are the experts in *you*. Physician decision making is not a "one shoe fits all" enterprise, yet when accurate, individualized information is lacking, that's what it becomes.

Whether you are startled by hearing a new diagnosis or you come to this knowledge gradually, learning that you have a neurologic problem is jarring. Many neurologic disorders are chronic; you aren't simply adjusting to something new—you will need to deal with this disorder for the foreseeable future. In certain ways, life has changed. Now, there are two crucial "next steps": the first is finding good neurologic care for your problem, and the second is successfully adjusting to living with your condition. This second step depends on attaining knowledge of your condition, learning new skills to manage the condition, and finding the flexibility and resourcefulness to restore your quality of life. When successful, you regain your equilibrium and restore a sense of confidence and control that is the cornerstone of well-being.

When healthy adjustment does not occur following a new diagnosis, a sense of feeling out of control and overwhelmed often persists, and no doctor's prescription will adequately respond to this problem. Individuals who acquire good self-management skills are often able to recognize and understand new symptoms and take appropriate action. Conversely, those who are lacking in confidence may respond to the same symptom with a growing sense of anxiety and urgency. In the first case, "watchful waiting" or a call to the physician may result in resolution of the problem. In the second case, the uncertainty and anxiety often lead to multiple physician consultations, unnecessary new prescriptions, social withdrawal, or unwarranted hospitalization. Outcomes can be dramatically different depending on knowledge and preparedness.

Managing a neurologic disorder is new territory, and you should not be surprised that you need to be equipped with new information and a new skill set to effectively manage your condition. You will need to learn new words that describe both your symptoms and their treatment to communicate effectively with the members of your medical team. You will also need to learn how to gather accurate information about your condition when you need it and to avoid misinformation. Although all of your physicians document your progress in their medical records, keeping a personal journal about your neurologic condition will help you summarize and track all your medical information in one place. When you bring this journal with you as you go to see your physician, you will be able to provide more accurate information about your history and previous treatment. Your active and informed involvement in your care and decision making results in a better quality of care and better outcomes.

Your neurologic condition is likely to pose new challenges in daily activities, including interactions in your family, your workplace, and your social and recreational activities. How can you best manage your symptoms or your medication dosing schedule in the context of your normal activities? When should you disclose your diagnosis to others? *Neurology Now*™ Books provide you with the background you need, including the experiences of others who have faced similar problems, to guide you through this unfamiliar terrain.

Our goal is to give you the resources you need to "take your doctor with you" when you confront these new challenges. We are committed to answering the questions and concerns of individuals living with neurologic disorders and their families in each volume of the *Neurology Now*™ Books series. We want you to be as prepared and confident as possible to participate with your doctors in your medical care. Much care is taken to develop each book with you in mind.

We include the most up-to-date, informative, and useful answers to the questions that most concern you—whether you find yourself in the unexpected role of patient or caregiver. Real-life experiences of patients and families are found throughout the text to illustrate important points. And feedback based on correspondence from *Neurology Now* magazine readers informs topics for new books and is integral to our quality improvement. These features are found in all books in the *Neurology Now*™ Books series so that you can expect the same quality and patient-centered approach in every volume.

I hope that you have arrived at a new understanding of why "knowledge is empowering" when it comes to your medical care and that *Neurology Now*™ Books will serve as an important foundation for the new skills you need to be effective in managing a neurologic condition.

Lisa M. Shulman, MD, FAAN
Editor-in-Chief, *Neurology Now*™ Books Series
Fellow of the American Academy of Neurology
Professor of Neurology
The Eugenia Brin Professor in Parkinson's Disease
and Movement Disorders
The Rosalyn Newman Distinguished Scholar
in Parkinson's Disease
Director, University of Maryland Parkinson's Disease and
Movement Disorders Center
University of Maryland School of Medicine

PREFACE

Navigating Life with Migraine and Other Headaches is written for those who have migraine and other headache types, their family members, and their caregivers. We have tried to write this guide in an approachable manner to give you a bit of background and understanding on what causes headaches and to address many of the questions that we frequently hear. We may not cover everything, but we hope this will be an informed start for everyone affected by headache.

This updated edition begins with a general overview and a discussion of causes. Did you know that Julius Caesar, Napoleon, Thomas Jefferson, Charles Darwin, Sigmund Freud, Vincent van Gogh, Pablo Picasso, and many other famous people had migraine? You're not alone! We've been trying to understand and treat headache for thousands of years.

Different types of headache are thoroughly explained in easy-to-understand language, beginning with migraine, which is the most common type of severe headache that can occur at any age. In children, it is more common in boys, but after puberty, it is much more common in girls. Even very young children are suspected of having migraine, although diagnosing them is almost impossible until they learn to speak. In women, it is most common between ages 40 and

45, while men tend to have migraine at a slightly younger age. This means that it often strikes people in their most economically productive years, which is a big part of the effect that migraine has on society.

We have included specific information about the different types of migraine: *migraine without aura* (previously called *common migraine*), *migraine with aura,* and other migraine types. Emphasis is placed on the necessity of early treatment, the importance of understanding the difference between a headache *cause* and a headache *trigger,* and how to avoid common triggers. *Rebound headache,* caused by the overuse of acute medication, is also a topic of special significance that is discussed in detail.

In addition to migraine, the book contains a chapter on tension-type headache, the most common primary headache disorder; 80 percent of us will have a tension-type headache at some time in our lives. Chapters describing cluster headache, unusual headaches, nonheadache illnesses that frequently accompany headache, sinus headache, disorders of the neck, post-traumatic headache, and atypical facial pain and trigeminal neuralgia are also included.

Treatment options for all types of headache are thoroughly discussed, including the treatment of migraine with medications that can be taken daily to help prevent headache, stop headache pain once it has begun, and prevent worsening of headaches. Different people have different responses to both prescription and nonprescription medications, so we cover this important topic as well. Managing your headache pain goes beyond simply popping pills; therefore, lifestyle issues are considered, including the possibility of depression or other psychological factors and family relationships. We've included information about alternative therapies, such as vitamins and herbal supplements, physical therapy, acupressure, massage, acupuncture, chiropractic care, craniosacral therapy, hydrotherapy, and yoga, as well as behavioral treatments, such as stress-management training and psychotherapy.

We hope that *Navigating Life with Migraine and Other Headaches* will help individuals with headaches, and those who care for them, to gain a deeper understanding of what is known about headache and what is *not* known, allowing them to explore diagnosis and treatment with this knowledge in hand. We are at the threshold of an explosion in the understanding, diagnosis, and treatment of migraine and other headaches, and soon more answers *will* be found.

William B. Young, MD, FAHS, FAAN

Stephen D. Silberstein, MD, FAHS, FAAN, FACP

Navigating Life
with Migraine
and Other Headaches

Section 1

Managing Your Headaches

Chapter 1

Introduction

Why Headache Is So Important

In this chapter, you'll learn:

- The scope of migraine as a public health problem
- How migraine (or chronic severe headache) affects quality of life

While driving home from work, Kathy was distracted by sparkling lights just to the left of her field of vision. When she turned to see what caused them, they moved away. She shook her head as if to shake them loose, and for a moment they disappeared. Within seconds, spears of bright light punctured the left side of her vision, too dramatic to ignore, and a tingling numbness ran up her left arm. She was concerned, but not frightened, until she looked down at the dashboard and couldn't read it because of a blurry patch in the center of her vision. She lived alone and had no one to call, so she turned left instead of right, and headed for the emergency department, tortured by fears of a brain tumor or some other medical horror. As she pulled into the hospital entrance, a stabbing pain seared through her left eye.

"You had a migraine," the neurologist told her, hours later, as she lay on the uncomfortable emergency department gurney, exhausted but finally, mercifully, pain free.

"All that from just a headache?" (Figure 1.1.)

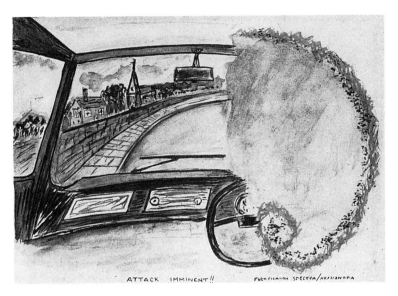

FIGURE 1.1 A patient's illustration of the migraine aura. Reproduced from Wilkinson M, Robinson D. Migraine art. Cephalalgia 1985;5:151–157.

Just a Headache

How often have you heard that phrase? **Headache** is such a common symptom that it often goes overlooked, undertreated, overtreated, or untreated. Actually, fewer people escape headache than experience a headache at least once in their lives. Although most people never see a doctor for their headaches, headache is the most common symptom for which patients see neurologists, and the seventh most common symptom for which they visit their primary care providers.

The impact of headache should not be taken lightly. Among chronic disorders, it is the third most common cause of missed work. It can affect you at home, at work, and in your interactions with friends and family members. It interferes with recreation, exercise, and the pleasures of everyday living.

Still, most people with headache self-treat or even ignore their headaches. Even people with **migraine** tend to put off seeking medical care. Despite the often-severe pain and other severely uncomfortable symptoms associated with migraine, reportedly less than half of sufferers consult a doctor for their problem. The reasons for this are many. Widespread misconceptions about headaches persist. Many people believe that "nothing can really be done" or that it is somehow weak to see a doctor for "just a headache."

In many ways, Kathy was fortunate. The odds of obtaining such speedy relief of symptoms are typically against a person experiencing migraine. The visual disturbances that startled her served as a warning, even more than the pain that followed, and led her to seek immediate help at an emergency department. Most people who have migraine do not experience an **aura** (see Chapter 3), the sparkling lights, numbness and tingling, and blurred vision that Kathy experienced. Still, many people, including some doctors, believe that without these symptoms, a headache cannot truly be called a migraine. When Kathy described her symptoms to the treating physician, she was referred to a neurologist. She was fortunate that the neurologist who treated her was knowledgeable about migraine and the latest treatments and that she was treated appropriately. She was also fortunate that she responded well to treatment. Even the newest and most appropriate treatment will not be effective in every case. The chapters in this book are aimed to guide you in your quest for better management and treatment of your headaches.

The Headache Experience

Greg thought his head was going to explode. A construction worker, he was a tall, heavily built man, attractive, with curly brown hair and hazel eyes. He was well liked and would often

(Continued)

(Continued)

cover for his coworkers. That was the reason he did not lose his job when he repeatedly called in sick. "A headache?" his coworker asked sarcastically when the foreman announced that once again they'd be short a man. "Jeez, Rob, we all get headaches!" He rolled his eyes. "This is the second day this week!"

"I don't know, Bill. Miriam said he was acting weird, pacing around the house, can't sit still. She's trying to get him to the doctor, but you know him—he won't go. She says she's worried, that one side of his face is all goofy. She thinks he's having a stroke or something."

Headaches can make you feel miserable. The quality of life for those with chronic severe headaches is very poor compared with that of people who have other disorders. Many, but not all, people with migraine have an extremely poor quality of life. Frequent absences from work and the inability to participate in many family and social activities are evidence of the extraordinarily negative impact that headache can have on your life. The significant decrease in your quality of life may even be severe enough to prompt you to seek care at a specialty headache center.

Headache and Your Family

"Be quiet, kids! Your mother has one of her headaches." From her bedroom, Angela heard her husband's voice in the hall. She had migraine attacks 2 or 3 days per month ever since she reached puberty. Every month her husband would darken the bedroom where she lay, keep the kids out of trouble and away from her, cook the meals, and run the house. He was a gem, her friends all told her. She was the luckiest woman on earth; if only she could feel well and enjoy it.

Headache Has an Impact

Migraine is a public health problem of enormous scope. Twenty-eight million U.S. residents have severe migraine. Of the people who have migraine, 25 percent have four or more severe attacks a month, 35 percent experience one to four severe attacks a month, and 40 percent experience less than one severe attack a month. Additionally, about 30 percent are severely disabled or need bed rest. Migraine is a lifelong disorder, but it may improve or worsen over time. Headache not only affects the person with headache, but it can also negatively affect family and friends. You may worry that at any time an attack will disrupt your ability to work, to care for your family, or to engage in social activities. Additionally, migraine is a condition that can have significant financial impact on you, your family, and your employer.

Headache has consequences on society. Inappropriate evaluation and treatment of migraine puts an enormous burden on an already overloaded health care delivery system. Migraine that is not correctly diagnosed and treated often results in an excessive number of unnecessary doctor office visits; frequent inappropriate emergency department visits; the overuse of unneeded and sometimes frighteningly sophisticated medical tests, such as magnetic resonance imagings (MRIs) and **computed tomography** (CT) scans; and the financial burden of purchasing inappropriate—and sometimes harmful—over-the-counter and prescription medications.

What You Can Do

Most of us who experience headache can be safely and effectively evaluated and appropriately treated by a headache specialist who has taken a detailed medical history and completed a thorough physical examination. The use of MRIs and CT scans is occasionally necessary for the proper diagnosis of a small number of headache patients. In other words, the time lost from healthy living, the absence from work, the expensive tests and inappropriate medications, and, in some cases, the resulting **disability** migraine causes are largely unnecessary and can be avoided with the proper tools and resources to manage your care!

Chapter 2

Pain, Disability, and Stigma
in Persons with Headache

In this chapter, you'll learn:

- That disparity exists between care and funding for headache compared to other neurologic disorders
- How disability associated with headache is underestimated and misunderstood
- How headache patients may be stigmatized by family, friends, colleagues, and even doctors
- How to help battle the stigma associated with headache through involvement in community action groups

Individuals with migraine rate their pain as severe or very severe almost two-thirds of the time. As discussed in Chapter 1, roughly 2 percent of the population has **chronic migraine**, and migraine is the seventh leading cause of medical disability, as measured in years of healthy living lost to disability. Additionally, migraine may have associated symptoms that headache patients find disabling, including nausea, vomiting, light and sound sensitivity, intolerance to motion and exertion, dizziness, and fatigue. The headache, accompanying symptoms, and resultant disability cause migraine to be one of the leading causes of days when patients cannot function fully at home, at work, or in society in general. Still, people with migraine are made to feel that it is unacceptable for them to take time off from their responsibilities. While people with migraine generally struggle through most of their attacks, it is common for migraine to affect work, self-care, and social and family life, completely transforming the type of life that headache patients can live.

In the United States, no criteria exist for migraine-related disability, despite the fact that specific criteria for neurologic disability exist for diseases with much lower impact, such as **epilepsy**. Appropriate evaluation by a headache specialist and treatment with lifestyle changes and medications that decrease, stop, or prevent headache pain greatly affect the patient's quality of life and ability to participate in family, work-related, and social activities.

What Is Stigma?

Stigma is the perception of a person's being less worthy than friends and colleagues, and stigma can mean the person is treated unfairly because of negative feelings toward people with the disease or condition. This devaluation of a patient's worth often is internalized by the patient, with resultant loss of self-esteem, confidence, and productivity.

> Tiffany has had near-daily migraine for 10 months. She has been given six different prescription medicines from two different specialists and still missed work on seven different days because she was vomiting and could not get out of bed. Her boss has mentioned that he has "concern" about her attendance.

The lack of attention to the disability of headache patients and the societal cost of headache cause the medical community to underestimate the significance of headache disorders as a life-altering disease with a high rate of associated disability. The National Institutes of Health funds **migraine research** at a level well below what would be dictated by its impact on medical costs, societal costs, and personal pain and disability. In fact, migraine and **cluster headache** (see Chapter 12) are the least funded of all neurologic diseases. Academic medical centers usually offer very little for patients with migraine, while they compete for the cancer patient, the **stroke** patient, and the dementia patient. When institutions are rated for their quality of neurologic care, they are expected to have a dementia center, a stroke center, a multiple sclerosis center, but never a headache center.

Doctors' prejudices can also stigmatize patients. Patients may feel their doctors do not recognize the legitimacy of their disease, sending subtle messages of disapproval. If a treatment fails, patients may feel blamed in a way that they would not if an antibiotic or chemotherapy failed. Some headache doctors have said that they do not believe anyone should be given disability for migraine, although loss of job due to migraine is not rare. People with chronic headache disorders are often heroic, carving out their best possible lives even if treatment has not been successful, and when work, friends, and family just do not understand. Having the confidence that you are coping in a brave and reasonable way can change your own perception of yourself and others' perceptions of you.

What Is to Be Done About the Stigma?

It is important for physicians, other medical personnel, hospital and insurance administrators, and laypeople to recognize the harm done by underestimating the pain, disability, and costs of inappropriately diagnosed and treated headache disorders. Prejudices against people with migraine who miss work, lose jobs, or fail to meet someone else's social expectations negatively impact the self-esteem, productivity, and social contributions of millions of headache patients. The medical and societal costs dictate more attention to migraine as a chronic disease and the need for funding of research and treatment centers. The good news is that government agencies, such as the National Institutes of Health, and professional organizations, such as the American Academy of Neurology and the American Headache Society, are working to overcome the negative perceptions of headache disorders.

A second important step toward getting understanding of headache and its treatment and having a positive impact on your community requires active involvement. Don't feel stigmatized. History shows us that disease-related stigma can be reversed when a community of patients comes together to raise awareness and funding for their cause. If you or someone you know has severe headache or migraine, here are some headache organizations that you can consider supporting:

- Miles for Migraine
- Runnin' for Research
- 36 Million Migraine Campaign/American Migraine Foundation
- Migraine Research Foundation
- Clusterbusters®
- Alliance for Headache Disorders Advocacy
- American Headache and Migraine Association

Chapter 3

Classification and Diagnosis of Headache

In this chapter, you'll learn:

- How primary and secondary headache types differ
- The importance of your headache history
- How the type of pain and other symptoms can help diagnose your headache type

Headache has many causes. It can be a **primary headache**, such as **tension-type headache** or migraine, meaning that the headache itself is the main medical problem. It can also be a **secondary headache**, a headache that is the result of an underlying medical condition, such as a neck injury or a sinus infection. Headache is rarely, however, the first sign of a dangerous medical condition (see Chapter 5).

Most headache patients have normal medical and neurologic examinations. When and how your headaches began provide important clues for diagnosis. Primary headaches usually begin in childhood or early adult life. However, if your headaches begins after the age of 55 years, a serious disorder is more likely. A headache that begins after a head injury suggests a **postconcussive** headache disorder or **intracranial pathology**, although head trauma may trigger both migraine and cluster headache. Fever in association with the onset of headache suggests an infectious cause. Exertion (e.g., weight lifting) may cause a harmless exertional headache, or it can precipitate a **subarachnoid hemorrhage**, an emergent type of stroke caused by bleeding into the space surrounding the brain.

Your Headache History

Where your head pain is located and the way it spreads help your doctor to make a diagnosis, because many headaches follow typical pain patterns. A unilateral, or one-sided, headache suggests migraine or cluster headache. Cluster headaches are always unilateral, with the pain centered in or around the eye. Headache of migraine can be on one or both sides of the head. On the other hand, tension-type headache pain is typically bilateral, and **trigeminal neuralgia** may cause pain in any area of the face.

Pain duration and other symptoms also provide clues for diagnosis. Migraine is typically throbbing, aggravated by movement, and associated with nausea, **photophobia**, and **phonophobia** (see below). It typically lasts from 4 to 72 hours. Cluster headaches usually last an average of 15 minutes to 3 hours. **Episodic tension-type headaches** (see Chapter 11) are typically dull and milder in intensity and tend to last from 30 minutes to 7 days. Understanding where your head pain occurs and how long it lasts is instrumental in helping your doctor diagnose—and ultimately treat—your headache condition (Table 3.1).

Clues for Diagnosing Your Headache

How often do your attacks occur, and what is the longest headache-free period you've experienced in the last 6 months?

- Migraine attacks may occur at random or in association with the menstrual cycle, on weekends, on vacation, or upon relaxing after stress.
- Episodic cluster headaches typically occur in a regular pattern. During the cluster period, which usually lasts between 2 weeks and 6 months, headaches may occur as rarely as once every other day or as often as eight times a day.

TABLE 3.1 Migraine or Tension-Type Headache

Characteristics	Migraine	Tension-type headache
Frequency	Variable	Variable
Duration	4–72 hours	30 minutes–7 days
Location	Unilateral (40% bilateral)	Bilateral
Description	Pulsating	Pressing/tightening
Intensity	Moderate–severe	Mild–moderate
Worse with physical activity	Yes	No
Nausea or vomiting	Yes	No
Photophobia or phonophobia	Yes	No
Aura	Yes (20%)	No

The attacks tend to recur at similar times of the day or night, and often wake the person during sleep.

- Episodic tension-type headaches occur fewer than 15 times a month. If they occur more frequently, they are classified as **chronic tension-type headaches**.
- Headaches of very sudden onset are worrisome. The headache of subarachnoid hemorrhage or pituitary apoplexy, both neurologic emergencies, typically have a sudden, explosive onset.

Pain is also a distinguishing feature:

- Migraine pain is characteristically throbbing or pulsating.
- Cluster headache pain is deep, boring, or piercing. It is sometimes likened to having a red-hot poker thrust into the eye.

- Tension-type headache pain feels like a tight band or vise around the head, and it can be mild to moderate in intensity.

When you get your headache, do other features come before, during, or after the pain? Do you experience other notable symptoms?

- Photophobia is an unusual or heightened sensitivity to light during a headache attack.
- Phonophobia is an unusual or heightened sensitivity to noise.
- **Osmophobia** is a heightened sensitivity to odors.
- Aura is a sensory perception (warning sign) before, or even during, a headache. It can be as mundane as tiny floaters in front of your eyes or as dramatic as hallucinations. The aura normally lasts about 20 minutes.

Understanding Your Headache

Headache has many causes. Most headaches are primary headaches, especially tension-type headache or migraine. Much less commonly, the headache is a secondary headache, due to an underlying medical condition, such as a neck injury or a sinus infection. Some people seek medical attention primarily because they are concerned that the headache is due to a serious underlying disease. MRIs and CT scans are rarely needed. However, more often, people seeking medical attention have severe pain and disability and require a program of care for improving their lives. Making sense of your headache history is the key to your diagnosis and treatment plan.

Chapter 4

Managing Headaches

In this chapter, you'll learn:

- What to bring to your first headache appointment
- What expectations of treatment are realistic
- How to partner with your doctor to treat your headache
- How to find a headache specialist
- How to work with your insurance company

What to Bring to Your First Headache Appointment

DOCTOR (TO COLLEAGUE): *"This patient never does what I suggest."*
PATIENT (TO FRIEND): *"The doctor just doesn't understand or care."*

If you have a burst appendix, your physician must take charge and direct treatment, and you take on a more passive role until it is time to recuperate. **Headache treatment** should *not* be like this. Headache treatment should be a two-way street, with you communicating your goals and desires regarding your headache management and your doctor bringing medical expertise and expectations, and both of you together developing a final treatment plan that incorporates both perspectives.

You may arrive at the doctor's office expecting an immediate diagnosis and rapid treatment and cure. Our recommendation is to have more realistic expectations. Diagnosing—and more important—treating your headache can take awhile, so be patient and work with your doctor for the best outcome. A patient may say, "I spent all day there. I had a bunch of tests, I filled out a gazillion forms, and I don't feel any better!" Headache control takes time, and sometimes a good deal of trial and error. Tests will not make you feel better, but they will help the doctor figure out how to do so.

Part of the responsibility of a conscientious caregiver is to help you understand your headache by clarifying the problem while laying the groundwork for the job ahead. Your doctor or nurse should teach you what you need to know to be able to manage your headache safely and effectively at home. Your doctor may not—in fact, should not—try to explain everything at once. It is almost impossible to retain information if too much is given to you in a single visit. The information that may be explained to you early in your course of treatment (in the first or second visit) includes:

- The difference between primary headache and secondary headache
- The difference between a **benign** and an ominous headache
- The difference between a trigger and a cause of headache
- The type of headache you have and its biological basis

If you have a primary headache disorder, such as migraine, you need to know that limited testing will stop and treatment will begin. People with primary headaches often search endlessly for a cause of their headaches and end up dissatisfied. Once the testing is completed and no secondary headache is found, it is best to accept the fact that the headache is a primary one and cannot be cured. If it is a primary headache disorder, blame and anger are not helpful and can actually worsen your headache. You and your doctor need to roll up your sleeves and get to work, because while treatment may be simple and effective, it could require many trials before a suitable solution is found.

What You May Do

A necessary first step may be stopping overused pain medication. Patients with daily headaches often become upset when doctors make this suggestion. Patients may believe that the doctor thinks they are addicted, but there is a big difference between addiction and medication overuse. Sometimes, overuse results in what is called **rebound headache**, a headache caused by overusing over-the-counter pain medication. Addicts are usually trying to escape from society or emotional pain. In contrast, patients who are "rebounding" want to take care of their families, do their jobs, and be part of society. Thus, they begin the vicious cycle of taking more and more medicine to continue functioning. Rebounders must understand that even if their motivations are excellent, rebound is an unhealthy behavior. No matter how noble the reasons, rebound must stop.

Establish realistic goals: if you want your severe headache to be gone in 5 minutes, and you are dissatisfied with anything that works more slowly, you will probably never be satisfied. Once a migraine is moderate or severe, the best oral treatments have a one in seven chance of relief at 30 minutes and a three in five chance of relief at 2 hours. That means that six out of seven patients do not have relief at 30 minutes, and a much smaller proportion of them are actually pain-free at 30 minutes. Outcomes improve greatly if the headache is treated in the mild stage or if an injection is used (see Chapter 7). Also, no medicine will work every single time. For some people, treatment will be successful 95 percent of the time, for others, 80 percent of the time, and a few unlucky people may find that the best they can get is a treatment that works half the time.

Try to establish realistic expectations about side effects for both **acute treatment** (which stops a headache) and **preventive treatment** (which keeps headaches from occurring). Most headache medicines have side effects that depend on the medication used (see Chapter 7). You may have to tolerate side effects and work to minimize them. The doctor can choose medicines that have fewer or less bothersome side effects for you or even side effects that provide some benefit; for example, a physician might choose a medicine that would cause nighttime sleepiness for someone with insomnia.

If you have a primary headache, your headaches may be controlled and may even stop. In studies of preventive medication, only half of subjects get 50 percent or more relief from their headaches with the first drug they try. Some doctors often do better than this by individualizing treatment, but they may need to try several preventives. With preventive treatment, headache improvement may not be immediate; it usually begins in about 4 weeks and generally it takes about 8 weeks to know if the preventive treatment is fully effective. You may be asked to tolerate some side effects. To minimize dissatisfaction, you and your doctor can use helpful strategies, such as once-a-day dosing and medicating before bed if sleepiness or other side effects could be caused by the treatment. So do not give up. Old treatments often work, and new treatments are constantly being developed.

Your Doctor and You

You should make your preferences known to your doctor. For example, your worst headaches might only be treatable at the cost of sleepiness. Maybe you would prefer to bear the pain and stay awake; maybe you would prefer less pain and some sleepiness. Some people will take the pain and not the medicine, while others will accept the side effects to obtain the benefit. The doctor-patient relationship is a partnership. Family members can be helpful, but they are not critical members of the treatment partnership. The doctor will, as much as possible, deal principally with you, not your spouse, mother-in-law, or concerned neighbor. Interested family members may be invited—by you—into the doctor's office and allowed to ask a few questions, but it is usually inappropriate for them to give most of the history or answer most of the questions. (Obviously, this does not apply when the patient is a young child or is mentally or psychologically incapacitated.)

Take charge of your care as much as possible. Know your medicines, including how often you take them. Understand the parts of your treatment plan that do not use medicines and how to implement those therapies. This helps to simplify treatment and puts you in charge of your own health and life.

To improve the partnership, help your doctor by being prepared to answer the basic questions he or she needs to know to adjust your treatment. Your doctor needs to know how often you have headaches, how long they last, and the intensity of your pain. Other questions might include:

- When did you first start having headaches?
- Have your headaches changed?
- When do your headaches occur (e.g., time of day, before or during menstrual cycle)?
- Do your headaches come and go?
- How long does a headache usually last?
- Do you have a headache virtually every day?
- Are you ever pain free?
- Where do you feel pain—on one side of your head, on both sides, behind one eye, in the front of your head? Does the pain move from one spot to another?
- Does the pain creep up and get worse, or does it start suddenly?
- How does the pain feel—dull ache, throbbing, mild, or excruciating?
- What other symptoms do you have with your headaches?
  - Do you feel nauseated or vomit?
  - Do you have sensitivity to lights or sounds?
  - Do you have visual symptoms or numbness before or during the headache?
  - Do you get any warning symptoms of a headache?

- What medications have you tried, and did these provide any relief at all?
- Do you take any vitamin or herbal supplements?
- Do you get a headache when you skip meals or eat certain foods?
- Do your headaches follow physical activity, such as having sex or exercising?
- Have you noticed a connection between extreme stress and the start of a headache?
- Have you noticed anything that seems to make the pain worse when you have a headache?
- Have you had any kind of head trauma—a car accident or sports injury, for example?
- Do others in your family have headaches?

You should prepare for these questions and be ready to answer them to the best of your ability. Many patients find that keeping a **headache calendar** helps when trying to answer these questions. You *must* be honest about the extent of your headache disability and medication use! It is absolutely vital to eliminate confusion, so don't keep secrets from your doctor. Your doctor may use a standardized questionnaire, such as the Migraine Disability Assessment (**MIDAS**), to help determine the impact your headaches have on your life (Figure 4.1).

What does the MIDAS questionnaire tell your doctor? Referring to Figure 4.1, first add up your answers to questions 1 through 5. If the total is 5 or less, you have minimal or infrequent disability, often with low treatment needs. However, if you have infrequent, but severe and disabling headaches, you may benefit from aggressive treatment. If the total is 6 to 10, you have mild or infrequent disability and have moderate treatment needs. If the total score is 11 to 20, you have moderate disability and have urgent treatment needs. Finally, if the total is 21, you have severe disability and very urgent treatment needs. If

1 On how many days in the last 3 months did you miss work or school because of your headaches?	☐☐	days
2 How many days in the last 3 months was your productivity at work or school reduced by half or more because of your headaches? *(Do not include days you counted in question 1 where you missed work or school)*	☐☐	days
3 On how many days in the last 3 months did you not do household work because of your headaches?	☐☐	days
4 How many days in the last 3 months was your productivity in household work reduced by half or more because of your headaches? *(Do not include days you counted in question 3 where you did not do household work)*	☐☐	days
5 On how many days in the last 3 months did you miss family, social or leisure activities because of your headaches?	☐☐	days
TOTAL	☐☐	**days**
A On how many days in the last 3 months did you have a headache? *(If a headache lasted more than 1 day, count each day)*	☐☐	days
B On a scale of 0–10, on average how painful were these headaches? *(Where 0 = no pain at all, and 10 = pain as bad as it can be)*	☐	

FIGURE 4.1 Migraine Disability Assessment (MIDAS). Reproduced from Stewart W, Lipton R, Dowson A, Sawyer J. Development and testing of the Migraine Disability Assessment (MIDAS) Questionnaire to assess headache-related disability. Neurology 2001;56(Suppl. 1): S20–S28. doi: http://dx.doi.org/10.1212/WNL.56.suppl_1.S20

you fill out the MIDAS questionnaire and your score is greater than 5, you should see a physician. If your job is at risk due to headaches, some very aggressive treatments may be reasonable, and this type of questionnaire encourages these important discussions.

To appropriately discuss the effects of medications, you need to understand the difference between an acute medicine (which stops a headache) and a preventive medicine (which keeps headaches from occurring). You should know the limits of how much of your acute medication to take to prevent rebound; if you are treating a headache with medicine every day, eventually the headache problem is likely to become much worse.

What We Think About Our Health Matters

People look at their own health in terms of three areas of control, or things that determine their health. One is the extent to which the doctor is in control, the second is the extent to which you control your own health and take responsibility for lifestyle changes that will improve your outcomes, and the third is the extent to which random, chaotic factors affect your health. All three factors are important. Patients who view their health as principally determined by the doctor or by chance do not do as well as those who have a more balanced view of the concept of shared control, and of the concept of individual responsibility for being compliant with all medications, lifestyle changes, and regular follow-up visits as suggested by their doctor.

Patients with headache need structure and balance. For many headache patients, a structured world without extremes or variability is the ideal. You can control stress, but it is not realistic to expect to eliminate it completely. Exercise regularly, or try to. Moderate food and alcohol intake and make sure that each day includes pleasurable activities; in general, strive to have a balanced lifestyle. Practice some form of stress-reducing technique daily, such as meditation, journaling, breathing exercises, or yoga (see Chapter 8). These measures can guide you toward a less stressful lifestyle or at least help you move in that general direction. You have to take the lead in your lifestyle modifications. Your physician can help you understand the aspects of your lifestyle that may be contributing to your headaches, but you must make a realistic compromise between the ideal and the other demands of your life. Significant evidence indicates that stress, sleep deprivation, hormones, and weather (to some degree) can trigger headache. Evidence also exists for some, but not many, food triggers. The best-identified food-related triggers are monosodium glutamate (better known as MSG), alcohol, and fasting. Sometimes patients develop false but very firmly held beliefs about the role that food triggers play in their headaches.

These may be patients who have headaches nearly every day, making it nearly impossible to identify food triggers. Very rarely, patients will need to go on an elimination diet, in which nothing but boiled rice is consumed for a number of days. If this does not control the headaches, it is reasonable to assume that food triggers are not very significant. Regardless, trigger identification requires a good doctor–patient relationship.

Keeping a headache calendar can be very useful in tracking and assessing the effect that your lifestyle has on your headaches (Figure 4.2; see also page 61 for further guidance on headache calendars). Before seeing a headache specialist for the first time, it is an excellent idea to keep a headache calendar for a few months. Eventually, headache calendar maintenance may no longer be worthwhile, as most of the information it can provide has been identified. Some people give their headache calendar such extreme attention that the headache takes on a bigger role than necessary. What is most important is to record your headache frequency.

Smoking cessation and exercise are beneficial to headache treatment. Aerobic exercise is most effective, and exercise that causes an increased pulse rate should be done for at least 20 minutes, 3 to 4 days a week. Mechanical disturbances of the neck and jaw may worsen headache, and mechanical changes that relieve stress on the

September **2017**

Sun	Mon	Tue	Wed	Thu	Fri	Sat
	1	2	3	4	5	6
7	8	9	10	11	12	13
14	15	16	17	18	19	20
21	22	23	2̸4̸	25	2̸6̸	2̸7̸
28	29	3̸0̸				

October **2017**

Sun	Mon	Tue	Wed	Thu	Fri	Sat
			1	2	3	4
5	6	7	8	9̸	10	11
12	1̸3̸	14	15	16	17	1̸8̸
19	2̸0̸	21	22	23	24	25
26	27	2̸8̸	2̸9̸	30	3̸1̸	

FIGURE 4.2 Sample headache calendar.

neck (moving the computer screen or changing a chair at work) or jaw (not chewing gum) may be helpful. For those whose headaches worsen with aerobic or high-intensity exercise, walking can be very beneficial.

The Mind–Body Connection

There is a commonly held belief that a severe psychological problem, such as **depression** or **anxiety**, will make headache more difficult to treat. Stress is the most common trigger for headache, and **biofeedback** (see Chapter 8) and **relaxation** can be very helpful for stress relief. Some headache patients need medication and/or psychotherapy for depression or anxiety, or they simply will not get better. It does not matter if the headache itself causes the depression or the anxiety; once it has started, it needs to be treated.

Family Relations

Family relations can be an important part of the headache problem and of headache management. There should be a balance of support. Family and friends can either be overly involved in your disorder or underinvolved to the point of being neglectful. Sometimes family members will assume "It's just a headache," such as one they've had themselves (usually much less severe). In other families, overinvolvement in the headache problem does not allow the patient to take charge of his or her own care. The family may undermine the treatment by demanding further tests and studies when they are time-consuming, expensive, and counterproductive to the treatment plan. Support groups (see Appendix 2) can be valuable, and the headache patient can choose his or her own level of involvement.

Treatment Overview

Headache treatment can be divided into treatments that use medicine and those that do not. If you have rare headaches, you may not need more than one type of treatment. If you have a severe, significant headache problem, your doctor will probably want you to try different types of treatment. During an office visit, you and your doctor may discuss the types of treatment (see below). Together, you and your doctor can decide on medication or treatment changes and make a plan to review the effect of the changes at the next visit.

Examples of Headache Treatment Plans

Headache treatment plans may include the following:

- Acute headache medicine may include nonsteroidal anti-inflammatory drugs for moderate headache or **triptans** for severe headache
- Preventive headache medicine may include a slowly increasing dose of **topiramate** (up to 100 mg per day) or amitriptyline (10 mg at bedtime)
- Lifestyle or other changes may include vigorous walking 3 times per week, regular meals, and regular bedtime
- Mindful ways may include biofeedback with relaxation training and yoga

Is Your Doctor Skeptical About Your Headaches?

Always remember that a good relationship with your doctor is key. If you aren't happy or have concerns about your doctor, don't be afraid to find a new doctor. It may take awhile to find a solution to your headaches, so it's best to be comfortable and trusting from the beginning. Here are some signs that you need to find another doctor:

- Your doctor is confused or uninterested when you describe your headache symptoms
- Your doctor tells you that you have to learn to deal with your headache
- Your doctor does not answer your questions
- Your doctor rushes you and suggests a pain medication right away
- You believe that you would benefit from seeing a headache specialist, but you cannot get a referral
- You take over-the-counter medications almost every day, but your doctor does not suggest a plan for you to stop taking the medicines
- Your doctor tells you that she doesn't feel comfortable trying to diagnose and treat your severe headaches

How to Find a Good Headache Doctor

- Ask your friends and family, especially those who are headache patients, for recommendations and referrals.
- Call a friend who is a physician, nurse, or other health care professional in your area.
- Call a local medical center or university and ask for the doctor-referral service, then ask for the names of headache specialists in your area.
- When looking for a headache specialist, you can ask if the doctor:
  — Is board certified
  — Is well credentialed to specifically treat headache (doctors may now become certified in headache medicine by the United Council for Neurologic Subspecialities)

— Is a member of a professional headache organization
— Frequently treats people who have headaches
— Takes courses and participates in continuing medical education that keeps him or her up-to-date with new developments in the diagnosis and treatment of headaches
— Publishes papers on headache and teaches others about headache

Working with Your Insurance Company

Insurance companies may have rules about access to specialists, inpatient hospital care, and medicines that may be necessary for you to get control of your headaches. How do you manage this?

You can ask for a referral to a headache specialist. If your primary care physician gives you a medication for your symptoms and it doesn't work, followed by the same routine a second or third time, you probably need to see a specialist.

You can ask your doctor to send a letter of medical necessity to your health insurance company. For example, if your health insurance company limits the number of migraine pills it will pay for in a given month, your doctor may need to send a letter of medical necessity to the company explaining what has been tried, over what time period, what worked, what didn't, and why you need more medication.

Many insurance companies deny payment for biofeedback and stress management or have made their reimbursement for these services so low that there are no providers in their plans who have the training or inclination to teach these skills. This is a difficult problem, and you might have to "bite the bullet" and pay for these services out of pocket. Ask your mental health practitioner if he or she provides this type of therapy in a group setting at a reduced rate.

Chapter 5

Headaches Requiring Urgent
Medical Attention

In this chapter, you'll learn:

- Warning signs that indicate a serious headache
- Reasons to see your doctor about your headaches
- What serious medical conditions are associated with headaches

*"Oh my God! The pain! My head feels like it's going to explode!
I hope it's not a brain tumor!"*

Fears of **brain tumor, aneurysm,** or other unknown but serious consequences usually cross the mind when someone experiences his or her first severe headache. With all the media attention that dramatic diseases generate, it would be unusual if those thoughts did not enter a person's mind. Fortunately, dangerous situations are rare. Primary headaches (headaches that are themselves the main medical problem) greatly outnumber secondary headaches (headaches that indicate an underlying problem), and headache is rarely the first indication of a dangerous medical condition. When should you seek immediate help? Red flags are warning signs and help to identify serious problems (Box 5.1). Comfort signs (signs that you shouldn't worry) suggest that the headache is a benign primary headache (Box 5.2).

BOX 5.1 Warning Signs of Serious Headache and When to See Your Doctor

Warning Signs

- Sudden-onset headache (maximum pain at less than 1 minute)
- Stiff neck
- Symptoms of brain damage, such as weakness on one side of the body
- Symptoms of a new, generalized illness, such as fever
- A known serious disease that can involve the head or brain, such as acquired immunodeficiency syndrome (AIDS) or cancer
- Relentlessly worsening headache over days or weeks
- New headaches starting at age 50 or older

Other Reasons to See Your Doctor

- You feel so bad you cannot go to work or enjoy yourself.
- Your headaches last for days.
- Over-the-counter drugs rarely provide relief.
- Your headaches have changed—they are getting more severe and occur more often than in the past.
- You get headaches with exercise.

BOX 5.2 Comfort Signs

Long history of headaches
Typical clinical features
Family history of a similar headache
Typical treatment response
Menstrual exacerbations

The following sections present problems that often include some form of headache as a symptom and require immediate medical attention.

Aneurysm

One of the most serious problems in which headache is a symptom is called a subarachnoid hemorrhage. In a subarachnoid hemorrhage, bleeding occurs under the membrane that surrounds the brain, which can cause pain. A subarachnoid hemorrhage is usually caused by the bursting of blood vessels that have weakened walls. Prior to bursting, the weakend blood vessel walls create a bulge, or aneurysm. If the aneurysm bursts, blood rushes onto the surface of the brain. Sometimes the blood vessel that breaks is part of an abnormal tangle of blood vessels called a vascular malformation. The headache caused when a blood vessel breaks comes on very suddenly, like being hit with a baseball bat. Occasionally it comes on more slowly, but it still reaches peak intensity in less than 60 seconds.

Aneurysm bleeds are true medical emergencies. A significant percentage of people with a bleeding aneurysm die before reaching the hospital. Many will die or suffer a stroke even with the best care. Early diagnosis and, in some cases, early surgery can save lives and prevent future strokes. Unless the aneurysm is surgically clipped or a coil is placed within it through the artery, the person with an aneurysm has a significant risk of the aneurysm bursting and bleeding, perhaps fatally (Figure 5.1). If you have a sudden-onset headache, or have several closely related family members with headache, you should see your doctor.

Subdural Hematoma

A subdural hematoma is a blood clot under the lining of the brain inside the skull. It often follows minor head trauma and can cause

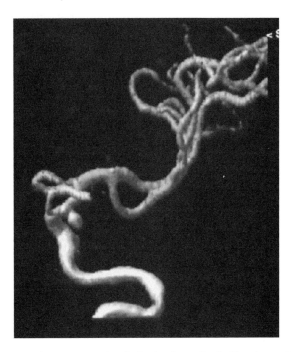

FIGURE 5.1 An aneurysm is a bulge in the wall of a blood vessel (*lower left*). This kind of image is used by neurologists to rule out diagnoses other than migraine. Reproduced with permission from Nitamar Abdala, Federal University of Sao Paulo, Brazil.

headache and neurologic symptoms, such as weakness or decreased consciousness.

Meningitis and Encephalitis

Meningitis is an infection of the cerebrospinal fluid and the linings covering the brain. There are several types of meningitis. The most dangerous form is *bacterial meningitis*, which is a critical medical emergency. A person with bacterial meningitis is usually very ill and has an extremely stiff neck, a severe headache, a fever, and sometimes reduced consciousness and seizures. Treatment with antibiotics should begin as quickly as possible, because long-term complications may be avoided with early treatment. People with viral meningitis are usually less ill and have fewer complications.

The headache in meningitis is usually felt on both sides of the head, is generally severe, and worsens relentlessly over hours or days. The neck is often so stiff that the patient has trouble bending the neck forward more than a few inches. The headache may be accompanied by sensitivity to light and sound, as well as nausea and vomiting. A mild jolt, such as hitting a small bump in the road while riding in a car, is extremely painful.

A person who has **encephalitis** has an infection that involves the substance of the brain, not just the coverings. Symptoms include reduced consciousness, weakness, severe dizziness, and speech and language problems, and they are more prominent than in meningitis. Meningitis and encephalitis require a **lumbar puncture**, or **spinal tap**, for diagnosis as well as a CT scan or MRI.

Brain Tumor

Headache caused by a brain tumor can resemble any type of primary headache but especially resembles a migraine or tension-type headache. A brain tumor can also cause worsening of a primary headache problem. However, headache is not the most reliable sign of brain tumor. More important signs of a brain tumor are symptoms like weakness, loss of vision, loss of sensation on one side of the body, clumsiness of the limbs, difficulty walking, and seizures; these symptoms are due to dysfunction of the part of the brain where the tumor is located (Figure 5.2).

Sometimes brain tumors present with a headache that starts out as mild, then worsens over days or weeks. This type of headache may also be caused by blood clots that press on the brain.

Hypertension

A common misconception is that headaches are caused by **hypertension**, or high blood pressure. For high blood pressure to cause
a headache, it has to be so high that it overcomes the normal protective reflex of the brain's blood vessels. While the point at which
this occurs varies, usually the **diastolic blood pressure** (bottom
number) needs to be above 115. Blood pressure that is so high it
causes a headache is a true medical emergency. More commonly,
headache pain may cause high, but not immediately dangerous,
blood pressure. Some blood pressure medicines can treat migraine,
and a headache may occur when a patient's blood pressure medicine,

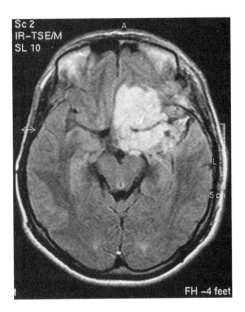

FIGURE 5.2 MRI is used in the diagnosis of several disorders of the
brain. This MRI shows a brain tumor (*circular light-colored area*) that was
the cause of headache and other neurologic symptoms. Reproduced with
permission from Suzana Malheiros, Federal University of Sao Paulo,
Brazil.

which also happens to be a helpful headache medicine, is stopped. Treating high blood pressure while also treating the headache gives the incorrect impression that high blood pressure causes headache.

Dissection

A **dissection** is a rupture of the lining of an artery. Blood enters and expands the wall of the artery, narrowing or completely blocking the artery and limiting blood flow to the brain. The headache from dissection can feel like migraine or **migraine with aura**. It may cause transient strokelike spells or a full-blown stroke. A stroke is a sudden loss of brain function that persists for more than 24 hours. Symptoms include weakness, numbness, blindness, and inability to speak (Figure 5.3).

Complicating this picture is the fact that people with migraine are at increased risk for developing a dissection. Minor neck injuries, including falls, car accidents, chiropractic manipulation, and even roller coaster rides, can cause dissection.

Spinal Headache and Other Low-Pressure Headaches

Lumbar puncture is a procedure in which a doctor collects cerebrospinal fluid through a needle placed into the lower back. This is a safe, minor surgical procedure with few long-term complications, and permanent injury is rare. However, about 10 percent of the time, a medium-term complication, called a **spinal headache**, occurs. This headache may be caused by a constant leak of cerebrospinal fluid through the hole made in the coverings of the spinal cord. The headache subsides when the patient lies down, and returns in seconds or minutes upon standing. It usually starts in the back of the head or upper neck and spreads over the entire head. Nausea and light and sound sensitivity usually do not accompany

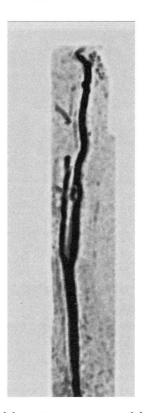

FIGURE 5.3 A carotid dissection is a rupture of the lining of the carotid artery that limits the supply of blood to the brain and can cause a headache that resembles migraine.

this type of headache. Lying down flat for hours after a lumbar puncture, the commonly recommended precautionary practice, does not protect someone from getting a spinal headache.

Spinal headaches almost always improve over several days. During this time, the patient should lie flat and drink plenty of fluids. Rapidly administered oral caffeine (No-Doz®) may also help, but intravenous caffeine is more effective. A procedure called a blood patch, in which the person's own blood is withdrawn from the forearm and injected into a space surrounding the spinal cord, may need to be done. This procedure is 98 percent successful and works instantly.

Section 2

Primary Headache Disorders

Chapter 6

Migraine

Causes and Triggers

In this chapter, you'll learn:

- The definition and types of migraine
- The symptoms and causes of migraine
- Some common migraine triggers and patterns

Definitions

"I've had headaches all my life," Keyanna said, sitting in the waiting room, "but they're not migraines."

"How do you know they're not migraines?" her friend asked.

"Well, with migraines, I read that you get a kind of warning. You know, flashing lights in front of your eyes and things like that."

"I sure do! I can always tell when I'm going to get a headache."

"Not me! It just hits me out of the blue. And do I get sick! My mother was the same way, and my grandmother, too."

When is a headache a migraine? Migraine is a process the brain and head goes through for which has no test. For years, even headache experts argued about what makes a migraine a migraine.

Finally, in the 1960s, a group of experts, "the Ad Hoc Committee on Classification of Headache," came up with a one-paragraph description of what constitutes a "migraine." This is what they came up with:

> Recurrent attacks of headache widely varied in intensity, frequency, and duration. The attacks are commonly unilateral (one-sided) in onset; are usually associated with loss of appetite and sometimes, with nausea and vomiting; in some [patients, they] are preceded by or associated with conspicuous sensory, motor, and mood disturbances; and are often familial.

For about 20 years, this was the accepted definition of migraine. Headaches that recurred, were usually one-sided, that sometimes seemed to cause an upset stomach, and were sometimes preceded by warning signals, such as flashes of light, dizziness, or changes in mood. By the early 1980s, doctors from the **International Headache Society** (IHS) decided that they needed a better way to diagnose migraine. They separated migraine into several types, the most common of which were **migraine without aura** and migraine with aura. (These had previously been called *common migraine* and *classic migraine*.)

Migraine without Aura

Keyanna, in our patient story above, probably had common migraine, or migraine without aura. The IHS defines migraine without aura as headaches that last for a defined period of time, usually hours. They have no known secondary cause and a neurologic examination is generally normal. The headache itself has to have some of the symptoms taken from the list below, but not necessarily all of them. In addition to pain, migraine needs to have nausea, with or without vomiting, and/or sensitivity to light and sound.

Description

The headache, when untreated—or treated, but without improvement—lasts from 4 to 72 hours. The headache is not caused by any other disorder.

At least two of the following characteristics are present:

- The headache is on only one side
- The headache is often described as throbbing
- The pain is moderate or severe and interferes with normal daily activities
- The pain is aggravated by walking up stairs or other similar physical activity

During the headache, at least one of the following is present:

- Nausea or vomiting
- Photophobia (sensitivity to light) and phonophobia (sensitivity to sound)

For years, migraine was referred to as a *sick headache,* and many people still use this term. This is most likely due to the nausea that occurs in over 70 percent of people who have migraine. Usually, migraine pain is aggravated by movement. Although migraine is thought of as one-sided, almost half of the time the pain occurs on both sides of the head. It often starts as a mild, dull headache, and as the pain becomes more severe, it starts to throb. During a migraine, many individuals are sensitive to light, sound, and odors.

Many people with migraine report sinus congestion or stuffiness. In fact, most people with a "sinus headache" actually have migraine; aside from congestion, imaging studies have shown that nothing is wrong with the nasal passages or sinuses in these patients. Many people with migraine report upper neck pain that can occur before, during, or after the headache pain.

> Mary first developed severe, one-sided headaches with nausea around age 14. Through high school, the headaches occurred a half-dozen times a year. By the end of college, they had increased to twice a month. Mary is now at her first job and is getting severe headaches three times a month. She also gets what she calls "regular" headaches. Aspirin works for the regular headaches but almost never helps the severe ones. Once a month, she misses work due to headaches.

Mary has migraine without aura. The headaches started a few years after her first period. They will probably be with her in various forms until after menopause. Since seeing a headache specialist, she has learned to take her prescribed acute medication as soon as she feels the headache coming on is usually able to head off the migraine. She also takes a preventive medicine every day, whether she has a headache or not. Her doctor prescribed 400 mg of vitamin B_2 daily, and she has noticed a decrease in the number of headaches. When she was asked to stop her high dose of B_2 while she was pregnant, her headaches increased again.

Migraine with Aura

Migraine with aura is the official name for a headache preceded by a physical warning of some sort, like something as mundane as tiny floaters in front of your eyes or as dramatic as hallucinations. The warning signs normally last about 20 minutes.

> On four occasions in the last year, Ronald experienced a concerning visual problem. He suddenly noticed a small spot that grew larger over the course of 20 minutes and then disappeared. The spot was surrounded by shimmering blue lights.
>
> *(Continued)*

(Continued)
He experienced this three times on the right side and once on the left. After the visual disturbance, a mild headache occurred, but it lasted only half an hour. He saw his family doctor, who found his neurologic examination to be normal.

Ronald has migraine with aura. Although his headache has unusual features—the headache is minor, the colored light is unusual, and the light portion of the aura is not very prominent—this could be little else but migraine aura.

Migraine with Brainstem Aura

Another type of migraine with aura is **migraine with brainstem aura**, also called Bickerstaff migraine. This type of migraine aura can include double vision, dizziness (vertigo), ringing in the ears (tinnitus), extreme unsteadiness in walking, and changes in level of consciousness or even loss of consciousness (fainting). This kind of migraine was thought to be more common in children, but it can occur at any age.

Stephanie, a 17-year-old girl, was in physics class when she had what her friends described as a "spell." Staring at the blackboard, she began seeing double. This lasted for about a minute. She began feeling as if the room was spinning, and then she passed out. Although her panicked friends insisted she was unconscious for at least 10 minutes, her teacher told the emergency medical technicians it was not more than 3 by his watch. When she awoke, she said her head hurt "terribly, all over," and she began to vomit. When she tried to walk, she was unsteady on her feet. This passed in a few minutes, but the headache lasted for hours. She was taken to the emergency department, where she was observed for several hours and discharged. Two weeks later, she had a second attack.

Stephanie has migraine with brainstem aura. This admittedly frightening syndrome causes no lasting problems, is nonthreatening, and, while it may occur several times, it is unlikely to be a severe problem. In later years, patients with this syndrome may develop other types of migraine.

The Cause of Migraine

For years, doctors and scientists have tried to discover the cause of migraine and offer relief. Over more than 100 years, many causes of migraine have been suggested, including nerve storms, vascular causes (related to blood vessels in the brain), an imbalance of chemicals in the brain that transmit signals from one nerve to another nerve, and inflammation of the membranes covering the brain and of the blood vessels of the brain. None of these suggestions has been supported by scientific research.

Currently, the best idea is the neurovascular theory, which suggests that migraine is due to an underlying brain disorder and increased sensitivity that affects the pain nerves inside of the skull that are known to be responsible for much of the pain of migraine. Migraine is much more than just head pain (Figure 6.1).

We have learned a great deal about what migraine is, but we do not have a complete understanding of the disorder, probably because migraine is not caused by any single factor.

The Five Causes of Migraine

We know five things about the cause of migraine, but there is no agreement on a single cause of migraine. It may be that migraine is not a singular problem but has multiple causes.

- Hypervigilant brain: The brains of people with migraine are hypervigilant and behave differently from the brains of people

CONTROL   **STIMULATED**

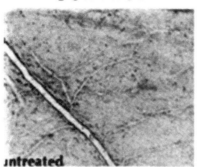 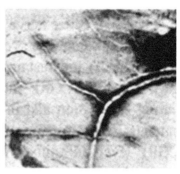

FIGURE 6.1 Blood vessels leak fluid during a migraine attack as a result of chemicals being released from nerve endings. Reproduced from Buzzi MG et al. Brain Research 1992;583:137–149 with permission from Elsevier Science.

without migraine. Scientific studies indicate that the visual part of the brain of people with migraine is more sensitive to certain kinds of stimuli and to repetitive sounds or visual stimuli. People with migraine show an increased response to repetitive stimuli, while people without migraine respond initially and then the response tapers off (Figure 6.2).

• Aura: The aura of migraine is caused by a wave of increased electrical activity that moves across the surface of the brain and is followed by decreased activity (Figure 6.3). The brief period of increased electrical brain activity is accompanied by a brief period of increased blood flow, then a period of decreased blood flow. This band of increased brain activity causes the bright lights seen in a typical visual aura. As the activated area travels across the brain, the person with migraine experiences a wave of bright visual hallucination.

• Brainstem activation: One or more areas of the brain that are specific for migraine turn on during a headache. One area of the brain in the upper brainstem is likely to be important

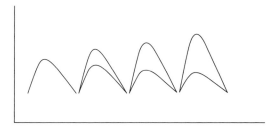

FIGURE 6.2 People with migraine are more sensitive to visual stimuli. The migraine patient's response to a series of visual flashes increases in intensity over time, whereas the response of a person without migraine to the same series of flashes decreases over time. Reproduced from Young WB, Silberstein SD. Migraine and Other Headaches (Fig. 6.3, p. 68), 2004, with permission from the American Academy of Neurology Press.

because it receives input from emotional and sensory areas and sends impulses back to these areas (Figure 6.4). Connections between this area of the brain and nerve fibers carry pain information into the brain. Connections with the pain centers receive information from the blood vessels in the brain.

- Inflammation inside the skull: Inflammation of blood vessels or the covering of the brain (the meninges) causes the throbbing pain of migraine. The nerve endings of patients who have migraine have been shown to produce an inflammatory protein called calcitonin gene-related peptide (CGRP) around the meninges and vessels. The blood vessels expand and the nerve endings on the blood vessels and meninges become more responsive, resulting in increased response to pain in these areas. This results in the throbbing pain of migraine.

- **Allodynia** (sensitivity to touch): People who have migraine attacks often develop sensitivity to normally nonpainful stimulation of the scalp, other parts of the head, and sometimes even the arm. This is called allodynia. Many patients with migraine experience scalp sensitivity and have increased

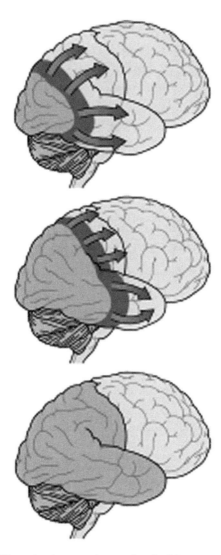

FIGURE 6.3 The migraine aura is associated with a wave (*black*) of increased electrical activity and blood flow followed by decreased electrical activity and blood flow. Reproduced from Lauritzen M. Brain 1994;117:199–210, with permission from Oxford University Press.

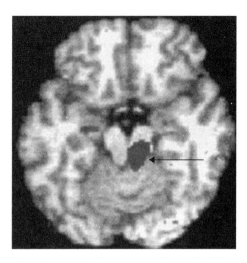

FIGURE 6.4 This positron emission tomography study shows blood flow changes in the brainstem during a headache. Blood flow increases (in the areas indicated by arrows) could cause the headache. Reproduced from Weiller C. et al. Nature Medicine 1995;1(7):658–660, with permission from the Nature Publishing Group.

pain when bending, straining, or shaking the head. Allodynia develops after the migraine starts; usually 1 to 4 hours later. Once it is established, migraine is much harder to treat because of increased brain activity.

Symptoms of Allodynia

- Tenderness of scalp
- Tenderness of muscles on head or neck
- Pain when brushing hair
- Aversion to cold wind through the hair
- Heat worsens headache
- Discomfort that causes patient to remove jewelry or loosen collar

Migraine Throughout Life

Migraine can occur at any age, including in young children and the elderly. Migraine tends to start earlier in boys (around age 10) than in girls (around age 15). Before puberty, it is slightly more common in boys than in girls, but after puberty, it is much more common in girls. Among women, migraine is most common between ages 40 and 45. Men tend to have a migraine peak at a slightly younger age. Migraine tends to strike people during their most economically productive years, contributing to the impact migraine has on society. In the United States, about 18 percent of women and 6 percent of men have at least one migraine attack per year.

In the elderly, the severe nausea associated with migraine tends to diminish. Also, aura is more likely to occur without a headache. These attacks can imitate a transient ischemic attack (TIA), which is a warning sign for a stroke. So, elderly persons with symptoms need to be evaluated by a physician at least once. Occasionally, hospitalization is needed to sort it all out.

Migraine Symptoms

To understand all the symptoms that migraine can cause, it is best to use the broadest definition possible, called *complete migraine*. The parts that make up a complete migraine include: the *prodrome*, the *aura*, the *headache*, and the *postdrome*.

The Prodrome

The prodrome occurs hours to 1 day before the headache and may involve a large variety of nonpainful behaviors and sensations. Typical symptoms include:

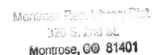

- Feeling sluggish or depressed
- Food cravings and increased appetite (and food cravings may explain why chocolate is often falsely identified as a trigger of migraine)
- Mood changes and often irritability
- Repeated yawning

The Aura

Aura occurs in about 20 percent of people with migraine. For some, it occurs with every headache, but more often it accompanies only some headaches. Many kinds of aura exist, but the most common is the visual aura. The most typical visual aura is called the *scintillating scotoma*. This aura generally starts as a small arc of flashing light just off the center to the right or left of the individual's area of central vision. Over about 20 minutes, a bright area of flashing lights expands to cover a significant portion of the visual field on one side. The bright lights are typically a pattern of short, flashing, and jagged lines. The lights are usually white or yellow, but they may be a variety of other colors. As the scintillation moves across the visual field, it may leave behind a scotoma, an area of decreased vision that is seen as black, gray, white, or clear. Visual migraine auras often vary from what is described above. They may occur on both sides of the visual field, travel from the outside to the inside, or even switch sides during a single attack. Patients often report that the visual problem is in only one eye. While it is possible that a visual problem originates in the eye (retinal migraine), this type of aura is rare.

The second most common type of aura is the sensory aura, in which tingling or numbness occurs for about 20 minutes. The numbness typically begins in one hand or near the lips on one side. It generally spreads or grows in the area of the body involved and may jump from the face to the hand or vice versa.

Migraine and Vertigo

In migraine with brainstem aura, the aura may be on both sides of the head and can lead to temporary blindness. This visual aura is often followed by ataxia (severe incoordination), vertigo, ringing in the ears, double vision, nausea, and vomiting. Jerky eye movements, slurred speech, pins-and-needles sensations on both sides of the body, or a change in level of consciousness and thinking can also be experienced. These changes usually last less than 1 hour and are generally followed by a headache. Although the symptoms can be upsetting, they signify nothing more than migraine with an aura clinically localized to the brainstem.

Other auras may involve *aphasia*, defined as the loss of the ability to speak normally, weakness on one side of the body, or a hallucination of an abnormal smell. One rare type of aura, more common in children than in adults, involves visual distortions and alterations in perspective and body image. It has been called the *Alice-in-Wonderland syndrome*, based upon the imagery in Lewis Carroll's novels.

Nicole, a 41-year-old woman with a long history of migraine, recalls peculiar spells during childhood. From the age of 4 to 17 years old, she would get "spells" entirely related to her hearing, "Every sound around me would assume the same overpowering rhythm." She eventually became accustomed to the spells and would lie down until they went away. Sometimes, particularly while reading, she would suddenly feel that her body had grown from the waist up; that she was looking down at the book from a distance of 10 feet or more. Another time, when she was riding her bike, she lost half of her field of vision. Her spells were not associated with headache. After age 20, she developed severe migraine without auras.

Michelle, a 23-year-old woman, has unusual seizurelike spells associated with her migraine attacks, occurring as often

(Continued)

(Continued)

as twice a day and lasting 20 minutes to 2 hours, but "Time is meaningless; it could be a second or days."

The right side of her face becomes numb and her tongue feels swollen, making it difficult for her to speak. Her eyes flutter and her balance is off. She has had at least one episode of confusion: while driving in the neighborhood where she grew up, she suddenly became disoriented, having no idea of where she was or how long the spell had lasted.

As a college student, Michelle experienced unusual spells. Once she woke up feeling tired and feverish; her temperature went from 99° to 104°F (40°C) within an hour. Four days later, she had a headache that she described as feeling like a volcano had erupted inside her head. Michelle was able to spell out numbers on her hands but could not speak.

The most striking episode occurred when a "little spaceman" took her into a "little spaceship." She could see her body lying like a dead weight on the bed beneath her; her mind and all that was essentially her floated in the air above her body. Her friend walked into the room, was unable to rouse Michelle, and summoned the campus emergency team. Michelle remarked that the static of their walkie-talkies pulled the spaceship back to earth when the ship attempted to "lift off." She was not frightened, but rather felt that she was in a "better place." When she awoke, everything was blurry; the movements and expressions of the people around her seemed both slower and exaggerated.

Nicole and Michelle have unusual migraine auras. Over time, and with repeated negative testing, the women themselves became certain their spells were all migraine.

Auras can occur one right after another. A person might first experience a typical visual aura, followed by a sensory aura, then an aphasic aura, and finally a motor aura. Some people experience a time gap between the end of the aura and the beginning of the headache.

The Headache

Following the aura is the next phase of migraine: the headache itself. Usually it is much like migraine without aura: throbbing, pulsating, or severe pain on one side of the head that gets worse with movement and is accompanied by nausea, vomiting, and increased sensitivity to light and sound. However, the pain can be on both sides of the head, and it does not always throb. Other symptoms may occur, such as pale, clammy skin and abdominal problems. Some headache patients vomit undigested stomach contents hours after their headache began. People with migraine may retain fluid during a headache, and their fingers, feet, and faces may appear slightly swollen. Thinking and behavioral problems may accompany migraine, such as difficulties with concentration and memory, decline in alertness, and a tendency to use the wrong word or to change letter order when writing. People with migraine usually exhibit "hibernation behavior" during severe headaches: they want nothing more than to crawl away into a cave.

Dizziness and lightheadedness are common during migraine, particularly during the headache. During a headache, a person may experience brief flashes of light called *phosphenes* that last seconds and may shoot or streak across the visual field, or they may experience allodynia. Many patients with migraine state that their "hair hurts," or that they cannot brush their hair during a severe attack, they dislike wearing jewelry or tight collars, and they avoid heat and cold applied on the scalp or air blowing on the head. This sensitivity usually starts near the site of the worst pain and travels to the other side of the head and sometimes down the neck to the arm.

Some people with migraine note that their headaches end in a distinct way. There may be an elimination of a large amount of urine, a bowel movement, or an increase in vomiting, followed by an abrupt sense of release of the pain in the head over the course of a few minutes. Some patients may induce vomiting with the intention of relieving severe headache.

The Postdrome

After the headache comes the postdrome, which often involves depression, weariness, or excessive joy. It can last hours to days. Preventing or treating the migraine early is the best strategy to manage this. No treatments are proven to be effective once the postdrome has begun, but it will go away.

Migraine Equivalents

Migraine equivalents are episodes that are very different from migraine and that occur without headache. The symptoms are not principally the associated symptoms of migraine. Yet migraine equivalents are not caused by injury and resolve like a migraine attack. Furthermore, at other points in their life, most of these patients get typical migraine.

At different ages, children may have repeated attacks that last hours or sometimes days. At about age 2, they may develop repeated spells of torticollis (neck twisting). Older children may get **abdominal migraine**, with attacks of stomach pain and vomiting that resolve completely. Adults may experience bouts of vertigo or dizziness that last for hours or days and then disappear spontaneously or respond to preventive migraine medication. This is called vestibular migraine. Older adults get auras without any headache or with only minimal head pressure. When an aura is not followed by a headache, it can be considered a migraine equivalent or it can be called migraine aura without headache.

Migraine Triggers

Common migraine triggers include menstruation, stress, relaxation after stress, fatigue, too much or too little sleep, skipping a meal, weather changes, high humidity, high altitude, exposure to glare or flickering lights, loud noises, perfumes or chemical fumes, postural changes, physical activity, or coughing. Food triggers occur in many adults with migraine and most often include alcoholic beverages (especially red wine), citrus fruits, and foods containing MSG, nitrates, and aspartate. Caffeine use and caffeine withdrawal may also trigger a migraine.

Menstrual Migraine and Other Hormonal Aspects of Migraine

Many women experience migraine as they enter puberty; the headaches generally improve after menopause. This pattern is related to the sex hormones **estrogen** and **progesterone,** which have an effect on migraine. Many women tend to get their most severe—or only—migraine attack around the time of their period. The most distinctive form of menstrual migraine occurs just after the onset of flow and appears to be due to the sudden drop in estrogen. Replacing estrogen just before and during the period reduces the occurrence of these attacks. The brain's abnormal response to normal hormonal fluctuations determines whether a woman develops menstrual migraine.

Some women have premenstrual migraine, or headaches associated with premenstrual syndrome (PMS). These headaches are often severe and may respond poorly to treatment. Menstrual headaches may be no more difficult to treat than other types of migraine.

In general, migraine gets better several years after menopause. However, some women report that their headaches worsen during menopause. Hormonal (estrogen) replacement may help this kind of headache, but many other factors need to be taken into account in any decision to replace estrogen after a natural menopause.

Migraine Patterns (As They Relate to the Clock)

Some patients have migraine that occurs at a specific time of day, time of month, or time of year. Early in the morning is the most common time for migraine to develop. Migraine may also start in the middle of the day and worsen in the evening.

Another migraine pattern has been termed *weekend headache*. Typically, a somewhat stressed worker will not have headaches despite a very active work week. On Saturday morning, the worker wakes up with a severe headache and is debilitated by nausea and vomiting. Three possible explanations exist for this phenomenon. One is that the release of stress has allowed the headache that was building up for several days to be expressed. A second explanation could be oversleeping; too much sleep may be a trigger for headache. The third explanation is caffeine withdrawal, since the first cup of coffee may come later on Saturdays than during the week. Keeping the weekend schedule similar to weekdays, especially waking hours and caffeine intake, may help.

Some patients have *seasonal headaches*, migraine that occurs only in winter or spring, for example. The causes of seasonal headache patterns are not known. They may be related to stress that is present only at that particular time of year or allergies or have some other neurologic connection.

Chronic Migraine

When migraine attacks become increasingly frequent, and the headaches occur on a daily or near-daily basis, they are referred to as *chronic* or *transformed migraine*. By definition, the headaches of chronic migraine occur more than 15 days a month, but they need not occur every single day. The less severe of the chronic migraine attacks often resemble tension-type headaches, with migrainous features becoming increasingly evident as the headaches become more severe.

Chronic migraine may evolve through a number of stages. At first, you may only have the occasional migraine, then the headaches become more frequent. The next stage is called *early chronic daily headache*, when the headaches are not daily, but occur more often than 15 days a month. Next, the headache usually occurs daily, but some hours are headache-free. The final stage is continuous, never-ending headache.

Chronic migraine, which affects approximately 1.5 percent to 2 percent of the population, has a more profound impact on quality of life than episodic migraine (migraine occurring fewer than 15 days a month). Chronic migraine pain may impact patients' ability to function, affecting their relationships with employers and coworkers, family, friends, and colleagues, and may lead to depression more often than in those who have episodic migraine.

Chronic migraine frequently develops in relation to overusing pain medications or acute migraine medication. This disorder was previously called rebound headache or analgesic-overuse headache, but it is now referred to as medication-overuse headache. However, the term medication-overuse headache is considered stigmatizing; hence many consider rebound headache a better term.

> Pat had episodic migraine for some time. The headaches occurred only four or five times a month, but they were so severe that he was missing work. His doctor prescribed Percocet. This worked well for him, and he was able to function well. So well, in fact, that he was
>
> *(Continued)*

(Continued)

promoted at work. With the increased responsibility came increased stress, and he noticed that the Percocet was no longer working as well as it used to. Sometimes he had to take two tablets. He called his doctor, who prescribed Fiorinal with codeine for the headaches that Percocet couldn't handle. This worked for a while, but it, too, became less effective. Soon Pat was taking some sort of headache medicine almost every day and often more than once a day.

Pat has medication-overuse headache. This occurs when an occasional headache develops into a daily, or almost daily, headache, and the medication that used to work no longer works as well. A medical or psychological stressor might trigger a bout of more frequent headaches. Needing to function, the patient takes headache medicine, but the need for medicine increases and so does the frequency of use. Eventually, higher doses of medicine and more potent types of medicine become necessary.

Linda developed occasional migraine attacks at age 13. By age 18, she had frequent tension-type headaches and monthly migraine. By the age of 25, she was taking Tylenol half the days of the month. At age 30, she was taking Excedrin three-quarters of the month. Now at the age of 35, she takes four to six Excedrin almost every day, Imitrex four days a week, and Fioricet 10 days a month. She misses 3 days of work a month and is there "in body but not in spirit" 4 or 5 days out of the month. She does much of the parenting of her two children while lying on the couch. She has seen two neurologists for her migraine and is dissatisfied with the care she receives.

Linda has a moderately severe case of chronic migraine with medication-overuse headache. Treatment for this complex problem involves medication withdrawal, use of an appropriate preventive medicine, and lifestyle changes that promote good headache control.

Mark had migraine without aura several times a month starting at age 6 and continuing into his teens and 20s. In his 30s, he took aspirin every day to prevent the headaches from getting bad.

In his late 30s, stress related to a car accident, financial difficulties, and helping to manage the affairs of his elderly parents resulted in his taking stronger narcotics. He was diagnosed with chronic medication-overuse headache, which upset him. He did not respond well to treatment because he did not follow the plan laid out for him by his headache specialist.

Mark has severe medication-overuse headache. He is not addicted, and attempting to treat him as though he were will probably harm him psychologically. Mark will need to be hospitalized to get off all pain medicines while being treated with dihydroergotamine injections to help with his withdrawal. The success of his treatment after hospitalization will require finding an appropriate preventive medication and explaining to him his responsibility to avoid medication overuse.

So how do you determine if you might be overusing acute medication? The most effective tool for this is the headache calendar (see Chapter 4). On it, you should note the time and severity of your migraine, what you took or did for it, and how well that worked. Examining the calendar, you should look for patterns of worsening or more frequent headaches, particularly severe headaches, within hours or days of discontinuing acute migraine medicines, an increase in the amount of medication you are taking, or preventive medicines or nonmedical treatments that previously worked well for you but no longer do.

Patients with medication-overuse headache may not have all of the expected symptoms. However, all of these patients need to see a headache doctor, who will put them on a headache preventive medication and possibly will suggest some lifestyle changes that are not medicine related. The effectiveness of such a plan depends on an agreement between the patient and the doctor that the patient will comply with the recommended plan and will not take any other pain or headache medications without consulting with the headache doctor.

Chapter 7

Treating Migraine with Medication

In this chapter, you'll learn:

- The difference between acute and preventive migraine medications and how each is used
- What kind of medications are used for migraine treatment
- The importance of early treatment

The most important thing that you and your physician can do to ensure success in treating your headaches is to keep the lines of communication open. Education about headache and its treatment is as important as any medication. When you receive a diagnosis, you should understand the implications of that diagnosis, what your symptoms mean, and what you can do to improve your situation. Your treatment plan should take into account your diagnosis, your symptoms, and your lifestyle.

This requires that you and your doctor share responsibility for improvement in your medical problem. Lifestyle changes to help manage your headaches, such as walking, getting a neck massage, or trying breathing and relaxation techniques at the first twinge of a headache, can all be effective. You have to be willing to put the recommended medication and lifestyle changes into action to achieve the improvement that you and your doctor are working for.

Exercise is good for your general health. It can reduce anxiety and tension, and it makes you feel refreshed. It may make you more flexible (especially if you stretch), condition your heart, and increase your energy level and ability to focus. Regular exercise, good health practices, regular mealtimes, sufficient sleep, and maintaining habitual patterns of activity are beneficial to people with migraine, because it is more difficult for these patients to adjust to unexpected changes in their daily routine. Hydration is also an important part of the lifestyle change.

Exercise increases your brain's production of endorphins, natural hormones that combat pain. Exercising three times a week for 30 to 45 minutes can help reduce headache frequency. Figure out which forms of exercise work for you and discontinue or change the ones that trigger headache.

It is best to follow a regular routine every day, with set times for going to bed, getting up, and eating. Additionally, you should not sleep in on the weekends. Avoiding or managing migraine triggers (see Chapter 6) can be effective, especially in combination with other therapies. Keep a record of the duration of your headache, its severity, its response to treatment, the medication you take for your headaches (including the dosage and what time you take it), and nondrug therapies. This information will be very useful as you and your doctor decide on possible changes or additional interventions.

Migraine: Acute Treatment

Acute migraine treatment acts to stop headache pain once it has begun and prevent it from getting worse. Two kinds of acute treatment may be used—specific and nonspecific. Specific treatments are for headache pain only. Nonspecific drugs work on other kinds of pain, in addition to head pain. They may work on nausea or other painful or inflammatory conditions as well as migraine (Table 7.1).

Which Acute Treatment?

Many acute treatment options are available—some are over-the-counter and some require a prescription. How does the person with

TABLE 7.1 Specific and Nonspecific Acute Migraine Medication

Specific	Nonspecific
Triptans	Acetaminophen (Tylenol®)
Almotriptan (Axert®)	Aspirin
Eletriptan (Relpax®)	Combinations of the above with
Frovatriptan (Frova®)	caffeine (Excedrin®)
Naratriptan (Amerge®)	Aspirin-free Excedrin®
Rizatriptan (Maxalt®)	Acetaminophen, isometheptene, and
Sumatriptan (Imitrex®)	dichloralphenazone (Midrin®)
Zolmitriptan (Zomig®)	
	Nonsteroidal anti-inflammatory drugs (NSAIDs)
Ergots	Ibuprofen (Motrin®, Advil®)
Ergotamine	Diclofenac (Cambia®)
Ergotamine and	Naproxen sodium (Aleve®)
caffeine (Cafergot®)	Many prescription NSAIDs
Dihydroergotamine	
Dihydroergotamine	**Barbiturates**
nasal spray (Migranal®)	Butalbital (Fiorinal®, Fioricet®, Esgic®)
	Opioids
	Codeine (Tylenol® #3, #4)
	Hydrocodone and acetaminophen (Vicodin®)
	Oxycodone and acetaminophen (Percocet®)
	Morphine
	Oxymorphone (Numorphan®)
	Hydromorphone (Dilaudid®)
	Butorphanol (Stadol®)
	Opioid-like medications
	Tramadol (Ultram®, Ultracet® [contains acetaminophen])
	Nausea medicine/neuroleptics
	Prochlorperazine (Compazine®)
	Promethazine (Phenergan®)
	Steroids
	Prednisone (Deltasone®, Prednicot®)
	Dexamethasone (Decadron®)
	Methylprednisolone (Medrol®)

migraine select the best over-the-counter medicine, and how does the physician select the most appropriate treatment?

One treatment may work for one individual, but not for another. Some, overall, are more effective than others. Acetaminophen is less effective, but has the least potential for stomach or kidney damage. Ibuprofen, naproxen sodium, and aspirin/acetaminophen/caffeine combinations appear to be more effective, but they have a higher risk of overuse.

By the time a person with migraine sees a doctor, it is likely he or she will have tried several over-the-counter headache medicines. Information on any medications or treatment you have had and how they worked goes a long way toward helping your headache doctor find the right treatment for you. Several factors are important in selecting a drug and how it is given: whether severe nausea or vomiting is present, how fast the medicine works, how severe the headache is, how long the headache has been present, the response to previous treatments, the side effects and safety of a particular medicine, and the chances of developing medication-overuse headache.

Studies have shown that treating a headache with the best drug for that attack is more effective than trying weaker medications and gradually working up to the right medication and dose. When patients are nauseated, antinausea drugs are indicated. If the patient is vomiting, nonoral preparations of medications, such as injections or suppositories, can be used. Additionally, injections can give much more rapid pain relief when needed.

Acute Treatment Types

Simple and Combination Analgesics and Nonsteroidal Anti-inflammatory Drugs

Simple analgesics, or pain medicines, are recommended for mild to moderate headaches. Many people find headache relief with simple analgesics, such as aspirin or acetaminophen (Tylenol®), either alone or in combination with caffeine, a well-established analgesic booster. Aspirin is not used in children younger than 15 years old due to the risk of Reye syndrome (see Chapter 9). We often try naproxen sodium is often tried first, but any of the nonsteroidal anti-inflammatory drugs (NSAIDs) can be used, often with an antinausea medication. Ibuprofen in over-the-counter doses is effective. Acetaminophen is as an alternative to aspirin or other NSAIDs for patients who have stomach inflammation or a bleeding disorder that prohibits the use of NSAIDs.

Barbiturate-containing medicines (Fiorinal®, Fioricet®, Esgic®) are still used. Because of concerns about medication-overuse headache, they should be used cautiously. In fact, these medicines have been removed from the market in many European countries, and patients taking these medications need to be carefully monitored. Nonetheless, they may be useful as backup medications when other migraine medications fail or cannot be used. For an individual attack, patients should take one to two tablets or capsules, with a maximum of six, per attack. The most frequent adverse reactions are drowsiness and dizziness. Drug use should be limited to no more than 4 days a month.

If nonopioid medications do not provide adequate pain relief, we occasionally use codeine in combination with a simple analgesic. We rarely use more potent opioid analgesics, such as butorphanol (Stadol NS®), meperidine (Demerol®), morphine, hydromorphone (Dilaudid®), and oxycodone and acetaminophen (Percocet®, Lorcet®), alone and in combination with simple analgesics. Because medication-overuse (see Chapter 6) are a risk with opioid use, opioids are most appropriate when severe headaches are infrequent and more specific medications (ergots or triptans) cannot be used.

Opioids should not be used more than 1 day a week, on average. Sometimes opioids are used more regularly for women with intractable menstrual migraine, but the risk of overuse is decreased since the headache improves when the menstrual period is over. Pregnant women can use codeine, but with caution. In susceptible

individuals, opioid use can lead to addiction. If your doctor prescribes opioids, he or she may inquire about the risk factors for
addiction: Do you have a family history of addiction? Are you under
great stress, highly impulsive, or sensation seeking? Have you been
exposed to physical, sexual, or psychological trauma or neglect? Do
you live in a social environment that makes addiction more likely?
Do you have other addictions, such as cigarettes or alcohol? People
who use opioids may be at a higher risk of death if they also use
benzodiazepines such as lorazepam (Ativan®), alprazolam (Xanax®),
or diazepam (Valium®).

Nausea Medicines and Neuroleptics

Nausea and vomiting can be as disabling as a headache itself. Some
nausea medicines are closely related to neuroleptics (antipsychot-
ics), and many are effective for headache, even if the patient does
not have nausea.

Delayed gastric emptying, or gastric stasis, a disorder that slows
or stops proper digestion and often accompanies a migraine attack,
decreases the effectiveness of oral medication. Metoclopramide
(Reglan®) is a nausea medicine that also stimulates normal gastric
emptying. Promethazine (Phenergan®) suppositories or ondanse-
tron (Zofran®) can be used by patients who cannot tolerate the side
effects of metoclopramide.

Chlorpromazine   (Thorazine®)   and   prochlorperazine
(Compazine®) are used intravenously (administered into the vein),
intramuscularly (administered into the muscle), and by suppository
(administered into a body passage or cavity) for nausea, vomiting,
and pain. Prochlorperazine suppositories are used as a primary
treatment for headache and nausea and as a rescue medication.
Giving a prochlorperazine injection intravenously or intramuscularly can be a therapeutic choice for migraine in the office or emergency department. Chlorpromazine is also available as an injection
or suppository, but the headache doctor most often prescribes it in

tablet form for a migraine "crisis" at home, to help ease pain and nausea and to allow the patient to rest.

Corticosteroids

Corticosteroids (prednisone, hydrocortisone, steroids, and dexamethasone [Decadron®]) are another type of headache treatment. It's possible they work in migraine by decreasing inflammation. They can be given intravenously, intramuscularly, or by mouth in tapering doses over a few days. Limiting their use to 5 consecutive days per month decreases the risk of long-term complications.

Ergotamine and Dihydroergotamine

Headache doctors rarely use ergotamine (Cafergot®, Wigraine®) to treat migraine. Triptans are now preferred to ergots for headache patients.

Dihydroergotamine (DHE) has fewer side effects than ergotamine and can be administered intranasally (through the nasal passage), intramuscularly, subcutaneously (under the skin), or intravenously. Nasal spray is not as effective as the other routes of administration, but it is well tolerated. Monthly use of DHE is limited to 18 vials or 12 events. DHE is useful because it is effective for most patients, is associated with a low headache recurrence rate (less than 20 percent), and is less likely than ergotamine to make nausea worse or to produce rebound headache.

Women who are attempting to become pregnant; patients with uncontrolled hypertension, sepsis, and renal or hepatic failure; and patients with coronary, cerebral, or peripheral vascular disease should avoid ergotamine and DHE. Nausea is a common side effect of ergotamine, but it is less common with DHE (unless it is given intravenously). Other side effects can occur, including dizziness, paresthesia (numbness and tingling), abdominal cramps, and chest tightness. Therefore, an **electrocardiogram** is recommended before the first dose of DHE, particularly if there are any cardiac risk factors or if you are over 40 years old.

Triptans

Sumatriptan is the most extensively studied agent in the history of migraine, but all triptans relieve headache pain, nausea, and light and sound sensitivity and restore the patient's ability to function normally.

You have an 80 percent chance of getting pain relief with a subcutaneous dose of sumatriptan and a 60 percent chance of getting pain relief with the oral triptans, but headache recurs about one-third of the time. Recurrences are most likely if treatment is delayed. Headaches respond well to a second dose of a triptan or to simple and combination analgesics.

None of the triptans should be used if you have a history of diseased cardiac arteries, Prinzmetal angina (chest pain), or uncontrolled hypertension (high blood pressure), or if you are at high risk for these conditions. Common side effects of triptan use include pain at the injection site, tingling, flushing, burning, and warm or hot sensations. Dizziness, heaviness, neck pain, fatigue, and mood changes can also occur. These side effects generally subside within 45 minutes. Chest pressure occurs in approximately 4 percent of patients. When patients are older than 40 or have other risk factors for heart disease, an electrocardiogram is obtained before a triptan is used. Other side effects—feeling medicated or fatigued, dizziness, weakness, and nausea—are common and may be severe enough to require an alternative treatment for future attacks.

Seven triptans are currently available. They are a safe (for patients without cardiovascular risk factors) and effective first-line therapy if you have a moderate to severe migraine or if pain medications have failed to provide you with adequate relief.

Headache severity, its rapidness of onset, and its duration are important factors that your doctor will consider when deciding which triptan should be used. When the headache intensifies rapidly (in less than 30 minutes) or nausea and vomiting are early and other severe associated symptoms are present, nonoral medications are appropriate. Subcutaneous injections of sumatriptan are the fastest and most effective treatment. Sumatriptan or zolmitriptan nasal spray may provide faster relief than oral triptans, but sumatriptan nasal spray is often associated with a disagreeable taste. Sumatriptan is now also available as an intranasal delivery system.

The oral triptans that your doctor may prescribe can be divided into two classes: those that work quickly and those that work slowly but have less chance of side effects. Almotriptan, eletriptan, rizatriptan, sumatriptan, and zolmitriptan are most effective quickly (within 2 hours), can provide headache relief within 30 to 60 minutes, and would be the first choice when you require quick relief and do not have multiple recurrences. Frovatriptan and naratriptan work more slowly but have fewer side effects (as does almotriptan). Almotriptan, frovatriptan, and naratriptan are choices for patients who are prone to side effects.

All triptans have the same contraindications and safety concerns. None is safer than another, however, and the response to triptans is often very individualized. One triptan may work for one patient and cause no side effects, while a different triptan may work for another patient. The triptan of choice is the one that restores your ability to function by swiftly and consistently relieving pain and associated symptoms with minimal side effects and without recurrence of symptoms.

Early treatment prevents worsening of pain and may increase the likelihood of relief. At least two attacks should be treated before deciding that a drug is ineffective. It may be necessary for your doctor to change the dose, formulation, or route of administration, or to add another medicine. When the response is poor, the headache recurs, or side effects are bothersome, you may need a medication change. All treatments occasionally fail; therefore, rescue medications, such as opioids, neuroleptics, and corticosteroids, are needed. They provide relief but typically limit function due to sedation or other side effects.

Over 73 percent of patients have nausea during their migraine attacks, while 29 percent of patients report vomiting during an attack. If these happen to you, tell your doctor, because nausea and vomiting are predictors of a poor treatment response to oral triptans. In addition, you may have gastric stasis (delayed emptying of the stomach) both during and between migraine attacks. This can slow absorption of medication and delay onset of benefit. If this happens, your doctor may consider medication that is not administered by mouth.

Treat Early or Late

Early treatment gets rid of your migraine more quickly and more completely than if you delay treatment. Early treatment also reduces the number of pills needed to treat each attack. If you treat too many attacks, you may be at risk of developing medication-overuse headache. Your doctor will work with you to develop an optimal approach for you, but for people with frequent migraine, the central tension of treatment is often balancing the effectiveness of early medication use against the risk of medication overuse.

Preventive Treatment

Preventive medications are taken whether or not headache is present to reduce frequency, duration, and severity of attacks. Preventive treatment can be preemptive, short term, or long term.

Preemptive treatment is used when patients have a known headache trigger, such as exercise or sexual activity, and a clear prodrome or aura symptom indicating impending headache (see Chapter 6). You should treat before the headache begins with a single dose of a preemptive medication. For example, single doses of 25 mg or 50 mg of indomethacin can be taken 1 to 2 hours before exercise to prevent exercise-induced migraine.

Short-term prevention (mini-prophylaxis) is used if there is an immediate risk of getting a headache, such as with menstruation, exercise, or high altitude. In other words, if you get headache from exercise, warm up slowly. Additionally, try taking ibuprofen or naproxen before exercise and be sure to stay well hydrated.

Long-term preventive medicines are taken on a regular basis (daily or at longer intervals for some injectable medicines), usually over months, to decrease the frequency of your migraine attacks. If you are pregnant, you should avoid preventive medications, unless severe pain or disability means the benefits of medication outweigh the risks. Circumstances that justify your using chronic preventive treatment include:

- Migraine significantly interferes with your daily routine despite acute treatment, and you have frequent headaches (more than one a week)
- Acute medications don't work, are contraindicated, are troublesome, cause adverse events, or are overused
- You preference (such as the desire to have as few acute attacks as possible)
- Special circumstances (such as prolonged migraine aura or attacks with a risk of permanent neurologic injury)

The major medication groups for preventive migraine treatment include beta-blockers, antidepressants, neuromodulating (or antiepileptic) drugs (NMDs), and NSAIDs. If preventive treatment is needed, your doctor will select a medication from one of these major groups, while taking into consideration the potential side effects and any coexisting conditions. Your doctor often will recommend that you start your preventive medication at a low dose. You can slowly increase the dose until the medication starts working, side effects develop, or the maximum dose is reached. Migraine frequently requires a lower dose of a preventive medication than what you would need for other medical problems. Try to remember that it may take 2 to 3 months to really get benefit. Medicine often does not start to work until it has been taken for 4 weeks, and benefits increase with time. It is not uncommon for someone to be treated with a new preventive medication for 1 to 2 weeks without effect and then discontinue it, based on the mistaken belief that it did not work. To obtain benefit from preventive medication, you should not overuse analgesics, opioids, or triptans. Migraine attacks may improve over time independent of treatment. If your headaches are well controlled, slow drug withdrawal can be started. Many patients experience relief after discontinuing the medication and may not need to resume treatment. Reducing the dose may provide continuous benefit with fewer side effects.

If you are a woman of childbearing age, you should use contraception before starting migraine medication. However, if you are pregnant, or if you are attempting to become pregnant, you may still require preventive medications. If it is absolutely necessary, you will need to work with your doctor to evaluate the risks and to pick the medication with the fewest potential adverse effects.

Medications

Beta-Blockers

Propranolol (Inderal®), metoprolol (Toprol®), timolol (Blocadren®), nadolol (Corgard®), and atenolol (Tenormin®) are all effective in treating migraine. Beta-blockers can produce behavioral side effects, such as drowsiness, fatigue, lethargy, sleep disorders, nightmares, depression, and memory disturbance. They are avoided if you have depression or low energy. Less common side effects include impotence, orthostatic hypotension (head rush), significant bradycardia (slow heart rate), and aggravation of muscle disease. Beta-blockers are especially useful for patients who also have chest pain (angina) or anxiety. They are usually not recommended for patients with congestive heart failure, asthma, Raynaud disease, and insulin-dependent diabetes.

Antidepressants

Many different types of antidepressants with different mechanisms of action are used in migraine prevention: nonselective tricyclic antidepressants (TCAs), selective serotonin reuptake inhibitors (SSRIs), and selective serotonin and norepinephrine reuptake inhibitors (SNRIs).

The TCAs (amitriptyline [Elavil®], nortriptyline [Pamelor®], and protriptyline [Vivactil®]) are commonly used for migraine and tension-type headache prevention. They are useful if you have trouble falling asleep. Side effects from TCAs are common and can include dry mouth and sedation. They can cause increased appetite, weight gain, and occasionally low blood pressure. In men with prostate enlargement, they can further hinder urinary flow.

SSRIs, such as fluoxetine (Prozac®), paroxetine, and sertraline, are used to treat **coexistent** depression, based on their favorable side-effect profiles and not because they are very effective, although fluoxetine may be effective in treating chronic daily headache. Some SNRIs (venlafaxine [Effexor®] and duloxetine [Cymbalta®]) are effective in migraine prevention. Sexual dysfunction is not uncommon with SSRIs and SNRIs, but it can be treated.

Calcium-Channel Blockers

Calcium-channel blockers are a type of blood pressure medicine often used to control migraine because of the mistaken belief that migraine is caused by changes in blood vessels. Verapamil (Calan®)

is the most widely used, despite limited evidence to support its use. Verapamil may be preferred to beta-blockers for patients who have high blood pressure and certain other conditions, such as asthma and Raynaud disease. Constipation and swelling of the legs can be side effects. However, low blood pressure is a less common side effect with calcium-channel blockers than with beta-blockers.

Neuromodulating Drugs

NMDs, or antiepileptic drugs, are increasingly recommended for migraine prevention because they decrease brain excitability. Divalproex sodium (Depakote®) was the first NMD shown to effectively control migraine. It is available in an extended-release form. The most frequent side effects are nausea, hair loss, tremor, fatigue, upset stomach, sleepiness, and weight gain. Rarely, liver problems and pancreatitis can develop. Before starting you on Depakote, your doctor will ask that your liver function be tested. If the results are normal, the liver function tests are not routinely repeated. The medication is not recommended in women of childbearing age because of the risk of birth defects.

Gabapentin (Neurontin®) is often used but is not very effective in reducing the frequency of migraine attacks. The most common side effects are dizziness or giddiness and drowsiness.

Topiramate (Topamax®, Trokendi®) is effective for migraine. It has been associated with weight loss, as opposed to weight gain, a common reason many discontinue preventive medicines. Side effects can include tingling, concentration and memory problems, kidney stones (rare), and glaucoma (even more rare). All of the side effects go away when the medicine is discontinued. Topiramate is often started at a dose of 15 to 25 mg/mL at bedtime and is increased weekly to 100 mg per day. (Of course, all dosages should be confirmed with your doctor, and you should follow his or her recommendations.) Topiramate may be taken twice daily, but taking it the full dose at bedtime is probably similarly effective.

Side effects often can be controlled by increasing the dose slowly and by keeping the maximum dose at 100 mg. Topiramate should be used with caution by patients who have a history of kidney stones.

Neurotoxin

Botulinum toxin (Botox®) is an U.S. Food and Drug Administration (FDA)-approved treatment for chronic migraine. The fact that Botox® can be an effective headache treatment was discovered by chance; patients told their doctors that their headaches improved when they were given Botox® to treat other conditions. This led to further investigation of its effectiveness for migraine, tension-type headaches, and other painful conditions.

How Botox® inhibits pain is under investigation. The injectable drug seems to prevent the pain associated with migraine, and perhaps other headache types, by getting into pain fibers and being transported backward to inside the skull. The effects of Botox® are long-lasting. It is given in a series of 31 injections every 3 months. Benefit increases for up to a year. The drug has no systemic or serious side effects; the most common side effects are temporary neck discomfort and possibly brow droop.

Special Circumstances

Menstrual Migraine

Many women get migraine and menstrual cramps with their periods. What can they do? First, consider the use of an NSAID, such as ibuprofen or naproxen, taken when the pain occurs or even on a daily basis (mini-prophylaxis). The triptans are effective for the acute treatment of menstrual migraine and can also be used for mini-prophylaxis. Many obstetricians/gynecologists have their patients take oral contraceptives for 3 months in a row without the pill-free week. (New oral contraceptives come pre-packaged this way and are now taken continuously.) They result in no menstrual periods and fewer headaches.

Exercise Headache

You may get headache from exercise. If this occurs, warm up slowly. Additionally, try taking ibuprofen or naproxen before exercise and remember to stay well hydrated.

Hospitalization for Headache

If you have chronic migraine with severe disability or uncontrolled migraine status, you may require hospitalization. The need for hospitalization may be suggested by the following:

- Not responding to aggressive outpatient treatments, including intravenous therapies
- Overuse of pain medicines, including barbiturates (such as Fiorinal® and Esgic®) and narcotics (such as codeine, oxycodone, and Percocet®)
- Severe desperation, up to and including risk of suicide
- Impending loss of job or withdrawal from school unless the headache is rapidly controlled

The goal is to restore function and to break the cycle of pain without painkillers.

Chapter 8

Alternative and Behavioral Treatments for Migraine

In this chapter, you'll learn:

- How to manage your migraine beyond taking medications
- The importance of lifestyle changes in migraine management
- How dietary supplements, physical therapy, and behavioral therapy can help manage your headaches

Alternative Therapies

Managing migraine, particularly chronic headache, means more than simply popping a pill. It is true that medication can do a great deal to relieve pain, but if you have a headache, particularly a chronic headache, you can benefit from an overall lifestyle plan that incorporates less traditional strategies. Along with appropriate medication, a properly balanced lifestyle, including a healthy diet, regular sleep, and some degree of exercise, will almost always reduce the frequency and severity of your headaches.

The goal of this chapter is to offer persons with headache an overview of the different therapies available and the potential advantages and disadvantages associated with each. For simplification, the treatments are classified as dietary, physical, and behavioral therapies.

Dietary Treatments

Dietary Supplements

Dietary supplements lie somewhere between traditional and non-traditional headache therapies. They are closest to traditional preventive medications in the way they are administered and the way they act. Most are vitamin, herbal, or botanical preparations.

Vitamins

Several vitamin supplements have been studied and found to be helpful in managing headache.

Riboflavin (vitamin B_2), at a dose of 400 mg/day, reduces the frequency of headache attacks and the number of headache days. It also improves the production of ATP, the molecule responsible for storing and supplying energy to our cells. Coenzyme Q similarly improves cellular energy production and has been shown to help migraine. Magnesium has also been studied and found to be effective in some studies and ineffective in others, but administered intravenously, it has shown potential for treating acute attacks.

Hydroxycobalamin, a form of vitamin B_{12}, also seems promising. It is a nitric oxide scavenger, and nitric oxide is thought to be involved in headache production. Hydroxycobalamin may be effective when taken intranasally, but more studies are needed to confirm this.

Pyridoxine (vitamin B_6) is used as supportive treatment for patients with histamine intolerance. The recommended dose is 100 to 150 mg/day. Check with your doctor before using higher doses, because they can be toxic. Histamine is believed to be involved in some cases of food- and wine-induced chronic headaches. People with histamine intolerance should follow a histamine-free diet. They should also avoid alcohol and certain drugs, as advised by their doctor. (If you aren't sure, or if you have questions, don't be afraid to ask about specific medications to avoid.)

Vitamins and botanicals can be harmful, especially when the dose is too high. Vitamin A is not a treatment for migraine, but its overuse leads to hypercalcemia and pseudotumor cerebri, a condition associated with severe chronic headaches, visual disturbances, and blindness. High doses of vitamins should not be used without guidance, and a balanced diet containing all the required nutrients is the best approach.

Herbs and Botanicals

Herbs and botanicals not only treat pain acutely but also relax and balance the body for longer-lasting benefits.

An oral extract of **butterbur** (*Petasites*) root (Petadolex®) has been tested as a migraine preventive with very successful results, but it has been removed from some markets because of liver toxicity. Another herb, **feverfew**, may also be effective, but the evidence has been conflicting and the herb is thought to contribute to medication overuse. Feverfew should not be used with warfarin, a blood thinner, because it may increase bleeding times.

Ginger is widely used to treat migraine, particularly in Ayurvedic (ancient Indian) medicine. It has not been proven to be effective for migraine, but it definitely relieves nausea.

Cannabis (marijuana) was used as a migraine treatment from 1842 until 1942. The first evidence of its use goes back to the year 5000 BC, with its first documented use for headache in the year 300 BC. Scientific studies have not shown a benefit from marijuana use for headaches, and there have been reports of marijuana being associated with both reduced and increased headache. The potential intoxicating effect, possible long-term harm with frequent use, and social stigmatization associated with this herb are likely to restrict its medicinal use in headache conditions. Ideally, better studies will allow providers to give accurate, scientifically based advice about the benefits and harms of marijuana use for migraine.

If you are pregnant, or thinking of getting pregnant, using high doses of most vitamins, minerals, or botanicals (Table 8.1) is not recommended. (The use of folate, a B vitamin, however, is strongly urged for all pregnant women and for all women of child-bearing age, to prevent birth defects.) The one exception is oral magnesium, which may prevent migraine but causes no toxicity other than diarrhea if the dose is too high in persons with normally functioning kidneys.

Physical Treatments

Physical Therapy

Physical therapy is used to strengthen neck muscles, to improve mobility, and to correct poor posture. Physical therapy can include heat (moist heating pads can be applied to ease pain and to improve mobility), ultrasound, massage for short-term pain relief, and strengthening and stretching exercises for long-term prevention of pain. Many people who have headaches have muscle tightness in the upper back and neck. Unraveling muscle kinks may help to relieve migraine pain. Cold is also used when areas are too tender to massage or stretch. Ice packs or vapocoolant sprays can be used. The sprays cool the skin and allow the therapist to stretch tender muscles with less discomfort.

The most commonly used treatments to stop a headache (acute treatment) are:

- Inhalation (using melissa, peppermint, and chamomile)
- Massage (with lavender, peppermint, anise, basil, or eucalyptus)
- Warm baths (with eucalyptus, wintergreen, or peppermint)

TABLE 8.1 Benefits and Harms of Vitamins/Botanicals/Herbs

Vitamin/Botanical	Benefits	Evidence of Harm
Butterbur	Migraine preventive	Liver toxicity led to withdrawal of government approval in some countries, including Germany
Cannabis	Migraine and tension-type headache	Tension-type headache with chronic use
Cocaine	No evidence of benefit	Brain hemorrhages (bleeding into the brain)
Coenzyme Q	Migraine preventive	Not known
Ephedra	Energy enhancer, weight loss promoter No evidence of benefit	Central nervous system toxicity (strokes, death)
Feverfew	Migraine preventive	Medication-overuse headache
Folate	Migraine preventive? No evidence of benefit	Not known
Ginger	Migraine preventive? Migraine preventive and abortive	Not known
Ginkgo biloba	Migraine preventive No evidence of benefit	Not known
Hydroxycobalamin	Migraine preventive	Not known
Kava kava	Relieves anxiety but not headache No evidence of benefit	Liver toxicity
Magnesium	Migraine preventive	Diarrhea
Passionflower	Sleep disorders? No evidence of benefit	None
Peppermint oil	Migraine abortive	None
Pueraria root	Migraine abortive No evidence of benefit	Not known

(Continued)

TABLE 8.1 Continued

Vitamin/Botanical	Benefits	Evidence of Harm
Pyridoxine (vitamin B$_6$)	Histamine-induced headache	Nerve damage
Riboflavin (vitamin B$_2$)	Migraine preventive	Not known
SAM-e (S-adenosyl methionine)	Migraine preventive	Not known
Tobacco	No evidence of benefit	Headache trigger Multiple adverse health effects
Vitamin A	No evidence of benefit	Pseudotumor cerebri, hypercalcemia
Vitamin E	No proven benefit	Not known
White willow bark	Acute treatment No evidence of benefit	None

- Compresses (of peppermint, vinegar, ginger, and marjoram)
- Others (e.g., herbal footbaths or headbands)

Cervical Manipulation

Cervical manipulation, movement of the neck by the therapist, is sometimes used to treat migraine. Maneuvers include mobilization, in which the therapist passively takes a joint or group of joints to the limit of the usual physical range of movement then returns to the starting point, and manipulation, during which a thrust is administered after the limit of the usual physical range of movement has been reached. Manipulations are done to increase the neck's range of motion and should always be performed gently. Neck manipulation carries with it an unlikely risk of stroke, so it should be used only as a last resort.

Acupressure

Acupressure is a finger-pressure massage targeting the acupuncture meridians, which are 12 invisible energy channels throughout the body used in traditional Eastern medicine. Shiatsu is a similar, but less intense, finger-pressure massage that targets the same meridians as acupressure.

Acupuncture

Acupuncture is a technique based on the flow of Qi Acupuncture, from Eastern medicine, is, the life energy force. Acupuncture is performed by inserting small needles into points along the meridians. Acupuncture is said to mobilize serotonin and norepinephrine, brain chemicals that block pain transmission and produce endorphins—the body's natural pain relievers. In some studies, acupuncture was not effective in the treatment of migraine and tension-type headaches. However, a recent study showed the benefits of acupuncture to be similar to those of an older antidepressant called amitriptyline. Many conventional physicians refrain from fully endorsing the use of acupuncture in migraine since few agree on how effective acupuncture is in treating pain. Acupuncture may be used as an additional therapy, because there is clear variability in response and no evidence of harm.

Chiropractic Care

Physicians have differing opinions on the use of chiropractic techniques for the treatment of migraine. Chiropractors use their hands to manipulate the spine to maintain a healthful balance. Neck manipulation should be avoided if you have, or are at risk of having, certain medical conditions, especially stroke. Some evidence exists that neck manipulations can, on rare occasions, cause stroke even in healthy people. Be sure to check with the headache doctor before receiving treatment and understand the risks this form of treatment carries.

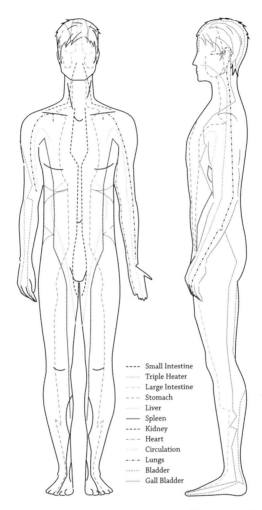

FIGURE 8.1 Acupuncture meridians (12 invisible energy channels) used in traditional Eastern medicine.

Craniosacral Therapy

Craniosacral therapy is based on a variation of osteopathic medicine, and its main principle is to increase the mobility of the bones in and near the head, reducing the pressure on the nerves of the skull and improving the flow of blood and cerebrospinal fluid. No studies have conclusively shown its benefit as a headache treatment, and success appears to be individualized.

Massage

Massage, either self-administered or given by therapists, not only is used by people with headache but also is effective in alleviating many forms of pain. Some studies show benefits of massage only during the actual therapy. The effectiveness of massage may differ depending on the type of headache. Nevertheless, massage helps to relax muscles, release the tension of tendons and other soft tissues, improve circulation, increase the uptake of oxygen, and stimulate the production of endorphins.

Hydrotherapy

Hydrotherapy is traditionally used as an adjunct to massage. It uses hot packs and ice packs, saunas, steam baths, and whirlpools.

Reflexology (Zone Therapy)

The principles of reflexology are similar to those of acupressure and shiatsu in that areas and points on the hands, feet, head, and ears correspond to other areas of the body. Applying pressure to or massaging specific areas enhances the well-being of the associated organs.

Qijong

Qijong is the skill of working with the "life force" by using movement and meditation to reduce stress, blood pressure, and muscle tension.

Yoga and Tai Chi

Yoga comes from the Hindu tradition and means to yoke, unite, or integrate. Yoga is not just a physical technique that stretches and strengthens but also a way of life that trains the body, mind, and emotions to unite with the spirit. The benefits of yoga are many, including increases in blood flow, relief of tension, release of endorphins, removal of toxins, and regulation of serotonin. The practice of yoga is highly recommended for headache patients and provides improvement in well-being even in people without headaches. When migraine is worsened by bending or yoga poses that put the head below the waist, tai chi may be an alternative. Tai chi is a noncontact martial art that is slow and performed in an upright position without any jarring movements. It has proven benefit for muscle pain.

Behavioral Therapies

Behavioral therapies are useful for persons with headache who prefer not to use drugs; who have trouble tolerating drugs; who are allergic to drugs or have other medical reasons to avoid drugs; who receive little benefit from drugs; who are pregnant, planning a pregnancy, or nursing; who have a history of excessive use of pain medications; or who have a psychological disorder, poor coping skills, or life stresses that aggravate headache problems. Behavioral treatments are often administered in small groups, allowing the cost of treatment to be reduced.

The goals of behavioral therapy include reducing the frequency and severity of headaches, lessening any headache-related disability, decreasing reliance on medications (particularly if they are poorly tolerated or unwanted), and improving personal control of headaches.

Behavioral treatments are classified into three broad categories: relaxation and relaxation training, biofeedback, and cognitive-behavioral (or stress management) training. Biofeedback and relaxation help patients who need to manage stress, especially children, pregnant women, and those whose headaches are brought on by stress.

Relaxation and Relaxation Training

Hypnotherapy is a kind of relaxation therapy that allows the participant to be highly receptive to suggestion. In 1958, it was approved by the American Medical Association as a therapeutic technique. Hypnotherapy has been shown to produce effects on the body similar to those produced by deep relaxation. In addition, a few studies show that it may decrease the frequency and severity of tension-type headaches and migraine.

Relaxation is considered the foundation and byproduct of many behavioral therapies and includes techniques that focus on breathing and relaxing your muscles.

The three most widely used types of relaxation training are: (1) progressive muscle relaxation—alternately tensing and relaxing selected muscle groups throughout the body; (2) autogenic training—promoting a state of deep relaxation by self-instructions of warmth and heaviness; and (3) meditation or passive relaxation—using a silently repeated word or sound to promote mental calm and relaxation. One study showed that after ten therapy sessions of progressive relaxation training, 96 percent of headache patients had a reduction in the frequency, duration, and severity of head pain. Deep breathing is often used in conjunction with relaxation techniques. With progressive relaxation, you take yourself through a series of toe-to-head muscle relaxation exercises. You start with your toes, contracting and relaxing individual muscles, then work your way up, gradually covering all muscle groups. This technique can also be combined with deep breathing. With visualization or guided imagery, you try to picture yourself pain-free in your own relaxing place—the beach, a boat, or curled up by the fireplace. Guided or unguided imagery and visualization can provide relaxation as well as direct effects on your body. Studies have shown that imagining a place or situation causes the same changes in the brain as if you were actually experiencing it.

Mindfulness meditation has data to support its use. It includes an awareness of what your experience is in the present moment with the intention of returning to the breath as an anchor when the mind wanders away from the present moment. Headaches may be associated with fear, and mindfulness is helpful in allowing negative emotions to be present without taking over and making the migraine worse than it has to be. Radical acceptance is a part of the practice of mindfulness meditation. It acknowledges the negative emotions associated with headaches while not allowing them to take over your essence.

Formal clinical studies of meditation have shown it to be effective in reducing pain, blood pressure, and heart rate. Changes in chemical blood levels in the body have also been reported. Many forms of meditation exist, and they all help patients to manage pain in addition to the stress of everyday life. Relaxation skills provide greater control over the body's responses to headache. Relaxation may also provide an activity break and help the individual gain a sense of mastery or self-control.

Biofeedback Training

Biofeedback is the most well-studied behavioral approach in migraine management and is proven to be effective. The technique is so well established as a preventive for migraine that some consider it to be a conventional treatment option. Younger patients and children in particular show many positive results from this technique.

In scientific studies, biofeedback has been found to be highly successful in migraine management. It is commonly used together with relaxation training, and the patient uses "feedback" from a body function to learn to control that body function. For example, hand warming, or thermal feedback, monitors skin temperature, and you learn to warm the temperature of your hands and feet. Electromyographic feedback monitors the electrical activity from muscles of the scalp, neck, and sometimes the upper body, and you learn to reduce the tension in these muscles (Figure 8.2).

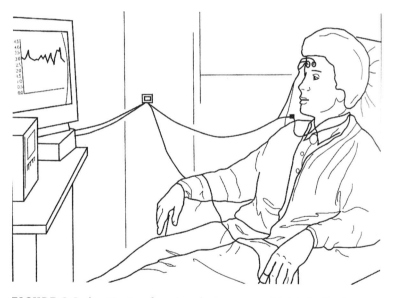

FIGURE 8.2 A patient undergoing electromyographic biofeedback training for frontal muscle relaxation as well as hand temperature biofeedback training. Reproduced from Young WB, Silberstein SD. Migraine and Other Headaches (Fig. 8.1, p. 116), 2004, with permission from the American Academy of Neurology Press.

Cognitive-Behavioral Therapy

Managing stress effectively is a useful skill for anyone, especially for a person with headache. Stress can bring on a headache, make it worse, or make it last longer. It can also increase the disability and distress caused by the headache. Learning to manage stress should be a priority in changing your lifestyle to reduce your headaches.

Stress management focuses upon the thoughtful and emotional components of headache. (Typically, it is used simultaneously with relaxation training.) It emphasizes the role our thoughts play in generating stress and the relationships among stress, efforts to cope, and headaches. With this technique, the patient is taught to use more effective coping strategies.

Some people with headache view their headaches as being outside their control or as the result of a personal deficiency. Either belief can lead to an attitude of helplessness. This need not be the case! You can monitor your physical reactions, thoughts, and emotional responses to headache-related stress. Relaxation skills can be used at any time. Self-regulation skills can be practiced in quiet, headache-free periods before being used to control physical responses throughout the day or to terminate some anticipated headache episodes. Audiotapes and treatment manuals can repeat and extend what is learned in treatment sessions.

Psychotherapy

Living with the pain and stress of a headache disorder can leave patients feeling helpless, frustrated, anxious, and/or depressed. These emotions can work against patients by worsening the headache condition by lowering their ability to tolerate pain and stress. Several forms of psychotherapy, or counseling, such as cognitive therapy, behavioral therapy, and support groups, can be helpful in dealing with the effects of disabling headaches. One study showed a major improvement in chronic tension headache patients involved in cognitive therapy. Support groups can offer a safe and understanding place to share struggles and feelings about one's headache disorder and can help patients feel less isolated. Some support groups can magnify hopelessness and frustration—those groups should be avoided.

Some Helpful Hints

Try to use simple ways of handling pain (walking, neck massage, breathing exercises, and relaxation techniques) before taking a pain-relief medication at the first twinge of a headache. Change what you are doing when a headache starts—take a walk or read a book. Distraction is effective for many mild headaches. Stop negative self-talk; replace negative thoughts with positive thoughts, such as "I'll feel better soon."

Chapter 9

Migraine in Children

In this chapter you'll learn:

- How headache in children differs from headache in adults
- How headache impacts the lives of children
- How headache in children may be treated

How Headache Affects Children

Children frequently have headaches, but they are rarely caused by eye problems, sinus infections, dental disorders, trauma, or food allergies. Similarly, brain tumors and other serious brain disturbances are very rare. Most headaches in children do not have a serious symptomatic cause except for a headache associated with a sudden fever.

The most common headaches in children are migraine, tension-type headaches, and headaches associated with an infectious illness. Headache affects the life of the child, can produce significant disability, and affects their families, including when staying home from school means their parents miss work. Most children and adolescents with headache never consult a physician.

- By age 3, up to 8 percent of children have had a headache
- At age 7, migraine occurs in about 3 percent of children and is more common in boys than girls

- Between the ages of 7 and 11, migraine occurs in about 10 percent of children and equally in boys and girls
- After age 11, more girls than boys have migraine
- By age 15, almost 82 percent of children and adolescents have had a headache

Jason had weekly bilateral headaches that prevented him from going out to play. He was sick to his stomach, and when he moved, the throbbing got worse. He is now 10 years old and has experienced these attacks for 2 years, but he is otherwise in good health. Jason has migraine.

Evaluating Children Who Have Headaches

If your child has headaches, your doctor will want to take a medical history from both you and your child. The history will include information about pregnancy, labor, and delivery, as well as your child's development, academic performance, behavior, and any previous neurologic problems. Does your child have sinus infections, abdominal pain, epilepsy, diabetes, trauma, or vertigo? Does your child use any drugs? The doctor may ask questions about balance, lethargy, seizures, vision problems, weakness, personality change, and trouble thinking. Are anxiety, tension, depression, nervousness, or school problems present? Recent exposure to fumes or toxins may be the cause of an obscure headache occurring only at home, so if your doctor doesn't ask, don't be embarrassed to share this information.

When headaches come and go without change and your child is otherwise healthy, it is most likely migraine. The doctor will do a complete general and neurologic examination, paying attention to blood pressure, height, and weight. The doctor will examine the skin and the skeleton for abnormal spots or evidence of injury. He or she will check the eyes for papilledema, or swelling of the back of the eye;

your child's head will be measured to rule out hydrocephalus (fluid in the brain), and the head and neck will be palpated for tenderness.

Children's migraine often goes undiagnosed because they have pounding headaches on both sides of their head and their headaches are shorter, lasting no more than a few hours. Kids—like adults— can have nausea and vomiting, light sensitivity, and dizziness.

If a child's headaches are increasing in frequency or changing in character, a new medical treatment should be suggested.

Features of Migraine in Children

Attacks are often shorter and occur on both sides of the head in younger children. As children get older, they develop one-sided headache. Children frequently experience nausea and/or vomiting with their headaches, with nausea becoming less frequent in older children. Children have an increased sensitivity to light and sound, with some having diarrhea, increased urination, sweating, thirst, edema (swelling), and tearing. Aura, when present, indicates that the diagnosis is migraine with aura.

Special Forms of Childhood Migraine

Abdominal migraine (recurrent abdominal pain lasting 1 to 72 hours) is a migraine equivalent. In this condition, a child has an attack of moderate to severe abdominal pain, commonly associated with loss of appetite, nausea, vomiting, or paleness, but without headache or head pain. Abdominal migraine occurs in 1 of 10 school-aged children. Often, the condition evolves into migraine, and many of the available migraine treatments (see Chapters 7 and 8) may be effective.

Hemiplegic migraine often starts in childhood and stops in adulthood. Attacks may be brought on by head trauma and usually last less than an hour. Typically, there is a visual aura, followed by the onset of slowly progressive one-sided numbness (or pins-and-needles sensations) and weakness. Difficulty with speaking and thinking of words and changes in consciousness are often seen. In rare cases, symptoms can last for up to a week.

Migraine with brainstem aura (formerly called basilar [brainstem] migraine) typically occurs in adolescent and preadolescent girls. Attacks usually last less than an hour and are usually followed by a headache. Common symptoms include trouble seeing or speaking, imbalance, vertigo, tinnitus (ringing in the ears), pins-and-needles sensations or weakness on both sides of the body, nausea, vomiting, and decreased level of consciousness.

Childhood periodic syndromes may be associated with migraine. They include **cyclic vomiting**, abdominal migraine, **benign paroxysmal vertigo** (dizziness), **alternating hemiplegia** of childhood (weakness or paralysis), and benign **paroxysmal torticollis** (spasms of the neck muscles). Other syndromes that occur in children include motion sickness, sleep disturbances (sleepwalking, sleeptalking, and night terrors), and episodes of unexplained fevers. The common features of these disorders are that they are recurrent, periodic, and associated with migraine or a family history of migraine.

Many children and adults with migraine will have a history of cyclic vomiting. Cyclic vomiting occurs in otherwise healthy infants and children, and children with this condition are likely to develop migraine. Cyclic vomiting is not unusual and is characterized by repeated episodes of severe, rapid-fire vomiting causing dehydration. Children are often pale and bothered by light. Cyclic vomiting occurs less commonly in adolescents and adults. Between the attacks, the child is completely healthy. Headache is not usually part of the syndrome. Preventive migraine treatment can be effective in decreasing the frequency and severity of attacks of cyclic vomiting.

Benign paroxysmal vertigo (intermittent episodes of dizziness) occurs in about 3 percent of children. Children develop sudden unsteadiness and grab on to whatever is near them for stability.

They stop all activities, appear frightened, refuse to move or stand, and have nausea and vomiting but do not faint. Nystagmus (jerky eye movements) may be present. The spell only lasts for a few minutes, and afterward the child may resume play or may want to sleep. The disorder often evolves into common migraine in later childhood and adolescence.

Alternating hemiplegia is rare and begins in infancy (onset before 18 months of age). The child has sudden, repeated attacks of weakness that involve each side of the body alternately and last hours to days. This is often associated with muscle contractions or spasms (**dystonia**). During an attack, the child is acutely uncomfortable. Alternating hemiplegia is a progressive disorder producing paralysis, developmental delay, and abnormal movements.

In paroxysmal torticollis, the child has attacks of involuntary twisting or tilting of the neck and head, vomiting, and loss of coordination of bodily movements. This can last from hours to days. Paroxysmal torticollis is a mild disorder that may appear frightening to an onlooker. It usually occurs in younger children, and it may evolve into more typical migraine later in life. The child often has a family history of migraine.

Secondary Headaches That Manifest in Children

A secondary headache is a result of an underlying medical condition, such as a sinus infection, brain tumor, idiopathic intracranial hypertension (a condition that occurs when pressure inside the skull increases for no apparent reason), or brain abscess (a collection of fluid that develops in the brain due to infection).

Brain tumors are rarely the cause of headache in children and adolescents. Most children with brain tumors experience chronic or frequent headaches. They are usually of recent onset and progress in frequency and severity and are associated with neurologic symptoms, such as seizures, weakness, and trouble thinking.

Idiopathic intracranial hypertension (also called pseudotumor cerebri) is increased cerebrospinal fluid pressure within the skull without evidence of an infection, mass (such as a tumor), or hydrocephalus (excessive fluid accumulation in the brain). Idiopathic intracranial hypertension is more common in adolescent girls. Patients usually have headache and papilledema (swelling in the back of the eye), double vision, and tinnitus (ringing in their ears). Lumbar puncture is needed for diagnosis.

Brain abscess is rare but may occur in patients with cyanotic congenital heart disease (a birth defect that can change the way the blood flows through the heart and lungs), chronic infections, or a reduction in the efficiency of a child's immune system from chemotherapy or human immunodeficiency virus (HIV) infection. Symptoms include fever, headache, weakness, and seizures.

Preventing Migraine in Children

It's important to remember that headache is generally considered a mild condition that most likely will improve within 6 months, independent of treatment. Because headache can be aggravated by stress, you'll want to modify your child's lifestyle to include a regular bedtime and a reasonable meal schedule and to avoid overloading of activities. Your child's doctor will also discuss various triggers that can lead to headache (e.g., physical exertion, hunger, noise, traveling, light glare, certain foods, and head trauma), and you should do everything possible to eliminate or avoid them.

Remember that the decision to use prevention depends on the frequency, duration, and intensity of the migraine attacks and the response to simple pain medication. Severe, frequent attacks often require preventive treatment. Migraine typically subsides after 6 months, particularly during summer vacation. If your child has been in remission for 3 or more months, your doctor may consider tapering and discontinuing the preventive medication.

Treating Acute Headache in Children

Treat early; the sooner you try to stop the attack, the better. Assure your child that it's okay to tell someone (including a teacher) when he or she is experiencing a headache. Use nondrug treatments when possible. When your child is experiencing an attack, have him or her sit quietly or lie down if possible; sleeping can help. Additionally, an ice pack or pressure on the painful area can be helpful. If medication is needed, consider over-the-counter NSAIDs, such as ibuprofen (Advil®, Motrin®) or naproxen (Aleve®, Naprosyn®, Anaprox®, Naprelan®). Acetaminophen (Tylenol® and others) may also be used for pain control. Aspirin should not be used in children or adolescents due to the risk of Reye syndrome, a rare condition that causes confusion, swelling in the brain, and liver damage. Aside from this restriction, children more than 12 years old can be medicated as young adults (see Chapter 7).

Chapter 10

Managing the Conditions that
Often Coexist with Migraine

In this chapter you'll learn:

- The definition of comorbid conditions
- The comorbid conditions that may occur with migraine
- The importance of managing comorbid conditions

Comorbid Versus Coexistent Conditions

Migraine is present in approximately 12 percent of people. Many other conditions can coexist and, in fact, are more common in patients with migraine. The conditions that have a more frequent occurrence in patients with migraine than would be expected by chance are considered **comorbid** conditions. Illnesses that occur in the migraine patient at a rate that would be expected by chance are called coexistent illnesses. All medical conditions that a migraine patient has affect migraine treatment. Common comorbid conditions associated with migraine that influence its management include depression, anxiety disorders, epilepsy, stroke, hypertension, and **obesity**. Sometimes, patients are misdiagnosed with another condition when the symptoms are actually those of migraine.

Allergy

It is uncertain whether allergies are more common in patients with migraine (comorbid). The uncertainty is caused by the fact that tearing, a runny nose, and nasal stuffiness are common during migraine attacks, and are often mistakenly diagnosed as **allergic rhinitis** (hay fever).

Stroke and Heart Disease

Individuals who have migraine with aura have a twofold increased risk of stroke, and the risk is even higher for women who smoke or use oral estrogen-containing contraceptives. Migraine with aura further increases the chance of heart attack and death due to cardiovascular disease, but it is not known why this is true. Some individuals with migraine can have numbness or weakness as part of their migraine attack; this does not mean they are having a stroke.

Epilepsy

Migraine and epilepsy are comorbid: if you have one of these disorders, you are more likely to have the other. The prevalence of epilepsy in the United States is 0.5 percent, or one out of every 200 people. If an individual has migraine, they have an almost 6 percent chance of having epilepsy. Similarly, 14 percent to 20 percent of individuals with epilepsy have migraine. The age of onset of epilepsy does not influence the risk of migraine. Persons with migraine with aura may have an even greater risk of epilepsy than those with migraine without aura.

Obesity

Evaluation for obesity is important in the management of patients with migraine. Weight gain is a frequent side effect of medications used to treat migraine. Obesity is a risk factor for increasing the frequency of migraine attacks, and both obesity and migraine are risk factors for stroke. No evidence exists that obese patients with migraine are more treatment-resistant than nonobese patients. Exercise, a healthy diet, and limited use of medications that produce weight gain should all be considered.

Pain

In some people, migraine may be comorbid with other chronic pain conditions. Children with headache are more likely to have persistent musculoskeletal pain. They are also more likely to have ear, shoulder, neck, back, and abdominal pain. This often leads incorrectly to the idea that migraine is due to neck or back problems.

Persons with **fibromyalgia,** a pain disorder that affects the muscles and soft tissue, have chronic, fluctuating, muscular-type pain in various parts of the body, such as the neck and the back. They also have tender muscles. Migraine, chronic migraine, and chronic tension-type headache are more common in people who have fibromyalgia. This may indicate that these disorders share a common overexcitement of the pain system.

Irritable bowel syndrome is another painful condition that is common in people who have migraine and vice versa. These individuals report recurrent abdominal pain, often alternating between constipation and diarrhea. Testing fails to reveal a cause of the pain.

Psychological Disturbances

What is the relationship between psychological disorders and headache? There is little to suggest a relationship with any headache condition except migraine, as it has been shown to be comorbid with depression and anxiety. Migraine is not a symptom of depression or anxiety, and most patients with migraine do not have either problem, but persons with migraine are three times as likely to have depression as those who do not. Similarly, anxiety and panic attacks are much more common in persons with migraine.

Surprisingly, it works the other way as well. Depressed people without migraine are more likely to develop migraine in the future than people who are not depressed. This relationship has been called bidirectional (functioning in two directions). Some people may have an underlying, perhaps genetic, predisposition to develop both migraine and depression. If someone has migraine and severe depression or anxiety, treating the headache alone will not be effective in relieving the pain until the psychological issues are also addressed.

Raynaud's Phenomenon and Autoimmune Disorders

When exposed to cold, the hands of a person with Raynaud's phenomenon become white, then pink and purple and very painful. Raynaud's phenomenon and migraine often coexist and may be comorbid for unknown reasons. Certain headache medications may worsen Raynaud's phenomenon. An increased risk of migraine also exists in individuals who have certain autoimmune diseases or disorders that cause pain and inflammation in the joints and connective tissue.

Restless Legs Syndrome

Restless legs syndrome is a condition that causes insomnia due to discomfort in the legs, and occasionally the arms, in the evening and when lying in bed. An irresistible urge to move the limbs accompanies these feelings. At its worst, the discomfort makes it impossible to stay in bed for very long before needing to get up and pace. The feelings in the legs and the need to move them make it extremely difficult to fall asleep. Patients often need to be completely exhausted so they can fall asleep quickly, before the need to move the legs and the uncomfortable feeling of restless legs syndrome make sleeping impossible.

Periodic leg movements during sleep can be very subtle but are sufficiently annoying to disturb sleep so that the deeper stages of sleep are never reached. As a result, an apparently normal amount of sleep is not restful in these patients. This condition overlaps with restless legs syndrome.

Restless legs are common in patients with migraine and fibromyalgia. They can be exacerbated by antidepressants and antinausea medications that are used to treat migraine. The syndrome is usually effectively treated by any of a variety of medicines taken in the evening or at bedtime. If sleep deprivation is making a headache problem worse, taking care of restless legs syndrome may be critical.

Managing Comorbid Conditions

Why is all this important? As a person with migraine, you are more likely to have one of these associated disorders. Patients with migraine and nausea are often given antinausea medicines, which can bring on restless legs syndrome and cause severe discomfort. Some migraine medications may worsen or cause depression. Others can result in weight gain.

Worsening of any other medical problem in a patient with migraine can have a serious impact. It is very difficult to control migraine with the presence of other untreated pain or with untreated depression. Be sure to maintain an open line of communication with your doctor so that he or she can help you manage your headaches and any comorbid conditions you may have.

Chapter 11

Tension-Type Headache

In this chapter, you'll learn:

- What tension-type headache is
- What causes tension-type headache
- How tension-type headaches can be treated

About 80 percent of people have tension-type headaches at some point in their lives. The headaches can last from 30 minutes to a week. The pain is a dull, achy feeling of tightness or pressure described as feeling like a band or a vise constricting the head. The pain is usually mild or moderate, in contrast to the moderate to severe pain of migraine. Sometimes the scalp, jaw, and neck muscles are tender, but patients do not have nausea, vomiting, photophobia, or phonophobia. Tension-type headaches do not usually interfere with daily activities, and physical activity normally has no influence on headache intensity. The stresses of everyday life aggravate tension-type headaches; therefore, they might be worse toward the end of the day. This is the headache most people mean when they refer to "just a headache."

Tension-type headaches can be episodic, when head pain occurs less than 15 days a month. Tension-type headaches can also be chronic, when headaches occur 15 or more days a month.

Causes of Tension-Type Headache

Some people who have tension-type headaches have scalp and neck muscle tenderness, but this is not believed to be the cause of tension-type headache.

Psychological studies of patients with tension-type headaches do not reveal any consistent findings either, although a few studies have shown higher levels of anxiety, depression, and suppressed anger in patients with tension-type headaches. In the most carefully performed study to date, it was concluded that people with tension-type headaches did not have more anxiety or other mood problems than people who did not have headaches.

When to Seek Help

So, when does "just a headache" become a serious enough problem to seek advice from a specialist? If your tension-type headache occurs more than 15 days a month, you have chronic tension-type headache. Chronic tension-type headache may be associated with medication overuse or rebound. Almost any pain medicine, including acetaminophen, can cause medication-overuse headache.

Some secondary headache types (see Chapter 3) have symptoms that mimic tension-type headache. If your headaches are of recent onset, the headache changes, or you experience neurologic symptoms, such as weakness, dizziness, or trouble thinking or talking, you should see your doctor.

Treatment of Tension-Type Headache

Episodic tension-type headaches are treated with acute medications. If the headaches are more frequent or become chronic, preventive medication is used, in conjunction with counseling, stress management, relaxation therapy, and/or biofeedback, as determined by the patient and the doctor together.

Medication

To stop or reduce the severity of an individual attack, the first choice is usually aspirin, acetaminophen, or ibuprofen, alone or in combination with caffeine, sedatives, codeine, or NSAIDs. Some doctors use muscle relaxants as well. The choice depends on the severity and frequency of the headaches, the associated symptoms, the presence of other medical illness, and your previous responses to medicine. If you require stronger medication, your doctor may suggest prescription medications and, in rare situations, prescribe medication that also contains butalbital, which causes sleepiness. Although these combinations may be more effective than simple pain medications, you should be aware of the high addiction potential associated with these drugs. Because of the risk of dependency, medication abuse, exacerbation of headache symptoms, or daily headache, analgesic overuse should be avoided. If you have concerns about any of these signs, be sure to contact your doctor immediately.

The major side effects of NSAIDs, including aspirin, are stomach upset, nausea, vomiting, constipation, ulcers, pain in the upper abdomen, diarrhea, and bleeding. Inform your doctor of any history of hypersensitivity to aspirin or any NSAID, a history of peptic ulcers, a bleeding tendency, severe renal (kidney) disease, or if you are being treated with anticoagulants (medication used to prevent blood clots). If you have kidney problems, you should also avoid these medications.

If the frequency and severity of your headache attacks warrant it, the doctor may suggest preventive medication, which might be an antidepressant, such as amitriptyline (Elavil®), the most commonly used preventive for tension-type headache, or fluoxetine (Prozac®). These medications have been shown to be very effective against headache, separate from their action against depression. Muscle relaxants may also be prescribed. Botulinum toxin (Botox®) is not effective for chronic tension-type headache.

Nondrug Treatment

You and your doctor may prefer to try nondrug treatments for your tension-type headaches, such as physical therapy. If depression, anxiety, or both accompany or aggravate tension-type headache, they are often the consequence rather than the cause of the headaches. Treatment may include biofeedback, stress management, and relaxation therapy, or cognitive-behavioral therapy.

Physical Therapy

Physical therapy consists of heat, cold packs, ultrasound, electrical stimulation, and improvement of posture through stretching, exercise, and traction. Physical therapy may be beneficial for patients who have tension-type headache associated with muscle spasm or tightness. Trigger point injections and occipital nerve blocks can also improve pain relief.

Biofeedback

Electromyographic (EMG) biofeedback enables patients to control muscle tension by providing continuous information pertaining to the state of tension of one or more muscles. An EMG sensor is used to provide a visual or auditory signal, allowing the patient to train the body to adjust muscle tension at will. Auditory feedback can be clicks or beeps that vary in rate, and visual feedback might be colored bars that vary in length. Sessions last about 1 hour. The treatment starts to work when patients learn to increase or decrease their head muscle activity. The ability to control muscle activity leads to relief.

Relaxation Training

Progressive relaxation training and autogenic training are both often used. Progressive relaxation training helps patients recognize tension and use relaxation techniques to reduce tension in everyday life. The patient learns to sequentially tense and relax various groups of muscles throughout the body. Daily practice of relaxation training at home is useful.

Autogenic training is a technique based on autosuggestion, and teaches your body to respond to your verbal commands. The patient seeks to simultaneously regulate mental and body functions by passively concentrating on a formula or mantra, such as "my forehead is cool."

Cognitive-Behavioral Therapy

The goal of cognitive-behavioral therapy is to teach patients to identify and challenge dysfunctional thoughts, with the intention of eliminating the negative thoughts. Cognitive-behavioral interventions, such as stress-management programs, may effectively reduce tension-type headaches, but they usually work best in conjunction with biofeedback or relaxation therapies, particularly if you have a high level of daily stress. These treatments have been shown to often improve the results of drug treatment.

Managing Tension-Type Headache

Tension-type headaches are the most common headache type. They are indistinct and usually not disabling. Most people have probably experienced a tension headache and used over-the-counter painkillers to treat it. Sometimes they progress to chronic tension-type headaches, especially when overusing medication. This requires more aggressive medical and nondrug treatment. Talk to your doctor if you require treatment for tension-type headache.

Chapter 12

Cluster Headache

In this chapter, you'll learn:

- What cluster headache is
- What causes cluster headache
- How cluster headache is treated

The term cluster headache refers to repetitive bouts of a specific and very painful type of headache over specific periods of time. These are cycles of daily, multiple, short-duration headaches that go on for 1 to 4 months and are separated by periods without headache attacks that last 6 to 24 months. Only 1 in 1,000 people is unfortunate enough to experience cluster headaches; of these, three-fourths are men, who are often smokers and are, or used to be, heavy drinkers.

Cluster headache attacks are one-sided. The pain is excruciating and located around the eye, temple, or upper jaw. It is often described as feeling like a hot poker in the eye. The attack can last from 15 to 90 minutes, occur one to four times per day, and often awakens the patient after 1½ to 2 hours of sleep. The attacks often occur at precisely the same time each day. The eye may water and become reddened, and the eyelid may droop. The face or eyelid may swell, and the nose becomes stuffy or runny on the side of the headache. While patients with migraine tend to be quiet and want to lie down in a dark quiet room, cluster headache pain may be aggravated by lying down. Patients with cluster headaches often become agitated and typically pace the floor, rock back and forth, or even bang their head against a wall during an attack.

Most patients have episodic cluster headache. If the attacks continue for 1 year without remission, the disorder is called chronic cluster headache.

Causes of Cluster Headache

The clocklike regularity of cluster attacks, with occurrences each day at particular times or in particular seasons, suggests that the disorder involves a part of the brain known as the hypothalamus, which functions as the brain's "clock." Recent neuroimaging studies using positron emission tomography (PET), an imaging method that allows your doctor to check for diseases in your body, show that the hypothalamus is activated during an attack of cluster headache. The agitated behavior during attacks may also come from this area of the brain. The pain is due to activation of the **trigeminal nerve**, which is responsible for sensation in most of the head and around the eye. The runny nose, sweating, and eyelid swelling are due to activation of a division of the nervous system known as the parasympathetic system. Swelling around the carotid artery behind the eye can damage another part of the nervous system called the sympathetic system. This can cause some people to have a droopy eyelid and small pupil on the cluster side.

Cluster Headache Experience

Mike, a 25-year-old smoker, had severe headaches when driving home after ending his shift at 4:30 PM. The headaches always occurred over his right eye, were excruciating, and lasted 1 hour.

(Continued)

(Continued)

His right eye teared and his right nostril was stuffy. When he got home, he could not sit still and would pace rapidly. His wife noted that his eye looked swollen and his whole eye was red during an attack. If she approached her husband, he would get angry and yell at her. By the weekend, Mike was getting two attacks; one in the afternoon and one waking him up 2 hours after he fell asleep. He also had an attack after drinking alcohol.

Mike went to the emergency department, where he was treated for migraine. After 2 months, the headaches went away but they resumed the next year, precisely on the day they had started the year before. This time, after just one headache, Mike went to the emergency department and refused to leave until he spoke to an expert. He finally got a diagnosis of cluster headache.

This story illustrates the severity and the clocklike regularity of attacks that many people with cluster headache experience. If the attack had occurred during work hours, Mike would have been unable to work while he experienced and recovered from the pain. Since his headaches occurred in the evenings, he had a good attendance record at work, but he was probably fatigued from lack of sleep and coping with his headaches. Mike's cluster attacks are typical for age of onset, presence of smoking, male gender, the number of attacks per day, and agitated behavior. However, Mike was fortunate that it took only 1 year to get an accurate diagnosis. It often takes several years before patients with cluster headaches are referred to a headache doctor who can diagnose this specific type of headache and recommend appropriate treatment.

Cluster Headache Treatment

Because of the incredible pain and the desperate awareness that the pain will recur, patients with cluster headaches need rapid and effective treatment. Before effective treatments were available, cluster headache was known as the **suicide headache**. The desperation is particularly severe in patients with chronic cluster headache.

Maintenance Therapy

Preventive treatment should be started as soon as possible in the cluster period. It may not be effective until the drugs have been used at sufficient doses for 1 or 2 weeks (Table 12.1).

Drugs that are commonly used for preventive cluster therapy, which are used either all the time or just when the cluster period is known to occur, include verapamil (Calan®, Verelan®), divalproex (Depakote®), and topiramate (Topamax®). Other possibly effective treatments include olanzapine and nasal capsaicin cream (capsaicin is a chemical extracted from chili peppers).

A surgical treatment that involves placing an implantable brain stimulator in the hypothalamus was developed to treat patients with chronic cluster who have very severe one-sided pain. Before this new surgical procedure, surgical interventions generally involved damaging the sensory nerve to the eye. The surgical procedures are reserved for patients for whom all preventive therapy has failed.

TABLE 12.1 Cluster Headache Preventive Treatment

Short-term Use	Long-term Use
Episodic Cluster Headache	Episodic Cluster Headache and Prolonged Chronic Cluster Headache
• Corticosteroids (prednisolone, prednisone, dexamethasone)	• Verapamil (sometimes a very high dose)
• Dihydroergotamine (DHE)	• Lithium
• Greater occipital nerve block with steroids	• Divalproex sodium
• Sphenopalatine ganglion block	• Topiramate
	• Melatonin

TABLE 12.2 Cluster Headache Abortive Treatment

Treatment	Effectiveness	Tolerability	Clinical Use
100% oxygen (7–12 L/min for 15–20 min)	Aborts headache in 70% in <15 min	Very well tolerated	First-line choice; inconvenient
Sumatriptan (20 mg intranasally)	Effective	Triptan side effects; contraindicated in cardiovascular disease	First-line choice
Sumatriptan (6 mg subcutaneously)	Highly effective		First-line choice
Dihydroergotamine (1.0 mg intramuscularly or intravenously)	Highly effective	Contraindicated in cardiovascular disease	First-line choice, but often hard to get
Lidocaine (4%–6% intranasally)	Questionable	Fair to good	Limited
Vagal nerve stimulator	Moderate	Excellent	Very recently approved; experience is limited

Transitional Treatment

Transitional treatment can be used to bridge the gap before preventive drugs take effect. Commonly used agents include corticosteroids and DHE. Corticosteroids (such as prednisone) provide rapid relief, and, while they are relatively safe in the short term, their long-term use may result in severe side effects, such as bone loss, muscle weakness, and increased abdominal fat. Repetitive intravenous DHE be used to break an attack of intractable cluster headache. An occipital nerve block containing a local analgesic and a corticosteroid is effective in about two-thirds of patients. Additionally, a nerve block for a group of cells accessible through the nose, the sphenopalatine ganglia, is now available in many centers and may be helpful.

Acute Therapy

Cluster headache may occur despite appropriate transitional or maintenance therapy. Acute therapies, used to shorten or stop the cluster attack, should be administered when symptoms begin (Table 12.2). They may resolve an individual cluster attack, but they will not prevent further attacks. One hundred percent oxygen, given for 10 minutes via a nonrebreather mask, is a safe and effective method of stopping a cluster headache attack. However, oxygen treatment often just postpones the attack. Sumatriptan (Imitrex®) and DHE are effective in ending cluster headache attacks, but their use should be limited to twice a day. DHE is the only medication that may stop the attack and prevent further attacks that day. Pain medicines, including opioids, are relatively ineffective.

A new handheld device, the vagal nerve stimulator, has just been approved for the treatment of cluster headache attacks. As of the publication of this book, there has been little clinical experience with it.

Chapter 13

Unusual Primary Headaches

In this chapter, you'll learn:

- What types of unusual primary headaches exist
- How unusual headache types may be treated

Unusual Headache Types

Several primary headache types exist that are much less common than migraine, tension-type headache, or cluster headache. These disorders need to be recognized and treated appropriately. They include **paroxysmal hemicrania, chronic daily headache, new daily persistent headache, hemicrania continua, ice pick headache,** and **sexual activity headache.**

Paroxysmal Hemicrania

Beverly was beside herself. Every day, over and over, she experienced 15 minutes of severe discomfort. She felt like her left eye and forehead were being stabbed with a spike. Her eye and nose felt like a slow leaky faucet. Then—suddenly—the pain was gone. On her best day, she experienced four of these episodes, but on her worst, it happened 30 times. If she took "tons of aspirin," she felt a little better.

Paroxysmal hemicrania is a very rare, clusterlike headache that mainly affects women. Like cluster headaches, the attacks occur only on one side, are centered on the eye, and are excruciatingly severe. They are accompanied by tearing, drooping of the eyelid, and facial swelling on the side of the headache. The major differences between paroxysmal hemicrania and cluster headache are that attacks are much shorter in paroxysmal hemicrania (15 minutes as opposed to 1 hour) and more frequent (usually more than six times a day). As with cluster headache, patients may have periods of remission without attacks, but they may also have be periods in which the attacks do not go away. Unlike cluster headache, paroxysmal hemicrania is well controlled by the medicine indomethacin (Indocin®). Because paroxysmal hemicrania has many similarities to cluster headache (one-sided, near the eye, eye redness, tearing, lid drooping, and running nose), the diagnosis may not be clear until indomethacin is tried.

Chronic Daily Headache

Unlike paroxysmal hemicrania, in which attacks of pain are short, chronic daily headaches are continuous or each attack lasts at least 4 hours. There are four types of chronic daily headache: chronic tension-type headache, chronic migraine, new daily persistent headache, and hemicrania continua. In these conditions, headaches occur on more than 15 days a month. (Chronic migraine and chronic tension-type headache are discussed in Chapters 6 and 11, respectively.)

New Daily Persistent Headache

Lori "never had anything but normal headaches," until a week before Christmas, 2 years ago when she woke up with a headache. She thought it was a tension-type headache, but it never

(Continued)

(Continued)

went away—not for a minute. When it was bad, she was sick, squinting in the quiet and just a little nauseated. She couldn't stop obsessing about the cause, and she had every test and an MRI and had seen an allergist. She vaguely remembered that her husband had a virus earlier in the month before her headaches started, and she was under the weather for a day and a half.

Diane, a 25-year-old woman, had few tension-type headaches until one morning she awoke with what she thought was another tension-type headache. By afternoon, she had a severe bilateral headache accompanied by light and sound sensitivity. She was unable to work for 3 days. Then, the headache decreased to the point where she had a daily headache, moderate in intensity and involving the whole head, with severe bouts of nausea and light sensitivity occurring twice a week. Over time, her symptoms increased until she began to miss work twice a month and rarely participated in optional activities. She had an MRI, a lumbar puncture, and many blood tests, all of which were normal, and she saw several specialists.

These are typical stories of new daily persistent headache, a subtype of chronic daily headache. New daily persistent headache starts suddenly and continues as constant, unrelenting pain. It is continuous, although eventually some people have headache-free periods lasting hours or days. People with this condition do not have a history of slowly worsening tension-type headache or migraine and can often pinpoint the exact day the headache started.

The cause of new daily persistent headache is unknown. No particular event can usually be identified, and brain imaging is almost always normal. In one-third of people affected, the headache begins around the time of a flulike illness. A virus called Epstein-Barr, which is responsible for mononucleosis, may be one cause. In one of eight individuals, new daily persistent headache starts around the time of surgery on some part of the body other than the head. Also, in one of eight patients, the headache starts at the time of a stressful event. It most commonly starts in the 20s for women and in the 40s for men; most people with this condition are women.

Many people with new daily persistent headache experience symptoms common to migraine: nausea, light and sound sensitivity, and pulsating head pain. A few even experience symptoms similar to an aura, including zigzag lines of light and numbness. Aggravating factors are similar to those for migraine and include stress, exertion, weather changes, bright lights, and menstruation.

No specific treatment exists for new daily persistent headache. It is treated as if it were the headache that it most resembles. If it has the symptoms of chronic migraine, it can be treated as a headache of migraine (see Chapter 6); if it has the features of tension-type headache, it is treated with the medications for tension-type headache (see Chapter 11). In general, new daily persistent headache is more difficult to treat than chronic migraine or chronic tension-type headache, but many people eventually improve significantly.

Hemicrania Continua

George developed a daily pain in his right temple and forehead. Sometimes he could almost ignore it, but it was always there, relentlessly aching. A few times a day, the pain got worse for about 10 minutes. His wife noticed his eye was moist and red during these times. She worried that he was taking too much over-the-counter ibuprofen, even though it didn't seem to help much.

Hemicrania continua is the least common of the unusual headache types. It is a continuous one-sided headache of moderate severity with periods of worsening pain. It may be accompanied by nausea, sensitivity to light and sound, tearing of the eye, eye redness, and a droopy eyelid during a severe flare-up. Some patients report a feeling of sand in the eye.

Hemicrania continua exists in both continuous and remitting (comes and goes) forms. The continuous variety can be continuous from the start or evolve from the remitting variety. The attacks of the remitting type last from 1 to 6 months, separated by pain-free periods of 2 weeks to 6 months. The cause of hemicrania continua is unknown.

Hemicrania continua, by definition, must respond to the medication indomethacin; therefore, for the doctor to make the diagnosis of hemicrania continua, the patient needs to try indomethacin. Unfortunately, some people cannot tolerate indomethacin because it causes stomach irritation and has a higher risk of kidney damage than other medicines in the same class NSAIDs. Occasionally, indomethacin makes people feel tired or generally ill. For these reasons, doctors and patients sometimes have to settle for another, often less effective, NSAID that has fewer side effects and fewer potential risks. Some patients have done quite well on the newest type of NSAIDs (COX2 inhibitors), particularly celecoxib (Celebrex®). Hemicrania continua may have features of chronic migraine, and, when indomethacin fails, it becomes chronic migraine.

Ice Pick Headache

Joan felt the most intense pain on the left side of her forehead, but seconds later, it was gone. It happened three more times that day and a couple of times after dinner. When the attacks continued into the following day, she urgently called her family doctor. Although her examination was normal, she was sure her doctor was missing something.

Some people get very brief, sudden, and severe jabs of pain with an onset that is almost instantaneous, but the pain usually resolves in as little as 1 second, although it may linger for as long as 30 seconds and occasionally a little longer. This kind of pain usually occurs in patients who are known to have another type of headache disorder, such as migraine or cluster headache. Occasionally it occurs by itself, and the patient has no other headache disorder. It usually is infrequent, occurring at most a few times a day. However, in rare instances, it occurs multiple times throughout the day and requires treatment with an NSAID, such as ibuprofen. The official medical term is idiopathic stabbing headache.

Despite the peculiar and severe pain associated with this headache, it is rare for any head or brain problem, such as a tumor, to be present. The pain is much too brief to be treated when it occurs, but it can usually be prevented by taking indomethacin, although it comes back as soon as the medicine is stopped. Usually only reassurance is needed; the pain is almost never a long-lasting or chronic problem.

Sexual Activity Headache

Headache can occur during sexual intercourse or masturbation. The most common type is an explosively sudden and severe headache occurring at or around the time of orgasm. This type of headache can be debilitating and last for hours. Because the nature of the pain is very similar to the headache that occurs as the result of a ruptured brain aneurysm, and since intercourse is a well-known trigger for rupture of a brain aneurysm, a person with a sexual activity headache should be very carefully evaluated to rule out a bleeding aneurysm. The evaluation usually involves a CT scan and a lumbar puncture, which should be done as soon as possible after the headache. If the patient is not evaluated within a few days of the headache, it may be necessary for the doctors to proceed with magnetic resonance angiography (MRA) or a more invasive test that involves inserting a catheter into the blood vessels that go into the brain. Most sexual activity headaches are harmless and can be treated once a dangerous aneurysm is ruled out.

The pain of the explosive form of sexual activity headache generally resolves within hours. It may or may not recur and sometimes occurs with each sexual activity. It can be prevented by taking indomethacin prior to intercourse. Migraine-preventive drugs are sometimes effective and must be taken daily.

Two other types of sexual activity headache can occur. One builds up slowly, has the symptoms of an exercise-induced migraine, and is treated as a headache of migraine. Another extremely rare type of sexual activity headache is a positional headache due to leakage of cerebrospinal fluid from a tear in the lining of the spinal canal, frequently following a lumbar puncture. Most patients improve spontaneously, although treatment sometimes involves finding the location of the leak and patching it with the patient's own blood taken from the forearm. If this is unsuccessful, then the tear may require a surgical repair.

Another severe condition, reversible cerebral vasoconstrictive syndrome, which is characterized by recurrent thunderclap headache (headache reaching maximum intensity in less than one minute) and sometimes neurologic symptoms, can initially resemble a sexual activity headache. If thunderclap headache is recurrent, one should consider the diagnosis of reversible cerebral vasoconstrictive syndrome, for which an MRA is needed.

Secondary Headaches and Neuralgias

Chapter 14

Sinus Headache and Nasal Disease

In this chapter, you'll learn:

- The symptoms of headache associated with rhinosinusitis
- How sinus headache and migraine differ
- How rhinosinusitis is diagnosed and treated

Rhinosinusitis and Headache

Acute **rhinosinusitis** is an infection of one or more of the cranial sinuses (air-filled cavities in the skull). Many migraine and tension-type headaches have symptoms similar to rhinosinusitis, and patients are often persistently, but incorrectly, convinced that they suffer from rhinosinusitis. However, frontal head pain is usually caused by migraine or tension-type headache, and nasal stuffiness is common in migraine.

The American Academy of Otolaryngology—Head and Neck Surgery changed the term sinusitis to rhinosinusitis because rhinitis, or inflammation of the nasal structures, typically comes before sinusitis. It is extremely rare to have infectious sinusitis without rhinitis. The tissues of the nose and sinuses are connected, and nasal obstruction and discharge are symptoms of sinusitis. The diagnosis of rhinosinusitis is usually based on symptoms related to the maxillary sinuses (located under the cheeks) or frontal sinuses (located under the forehead). Acute rhinosinusitis affects about 30 million people in the United States per year, and, according to data from the National Ambulatory Medical Care Survey, the problem is increasing.

In children, the most common sites of sinus infection are the maxillary sinuses and ethmoid sinuses, located behind the nose. These sinuses are present at birth. Other sinuses, located deep in the head, develop during childhood. The frontal and sphenoidal sinuses (in back of the nose) are frequent sites of infection among teenagers.

Cause of Rhinosinusitis

Obstruction of the entrance to the sinuses is the major cause of rhinosinusitis and sinus headache. The sinuses are air-filled cavities that connect with the nasal passages and warm and humidify the air we breathe. The cavities are lined with cells that contain hairlike projections covered by a thin layer of mucus. The hairlike structures move in a way that creates a flow of mucus out of the sinus into the nasal cavity. When this flow of mucus is stopped, a "stuffed up" feeling is often the result.

Testing and Diagnosis

Diagnostic testing to examine the sinuses for rhinosinusitis may include **computed tomography** or **nasal endoscopy**. CT is the best study to evaluate the sinuses, better than an MRI. A CT scan may show thickening of the surface of the sinuses, scarring, clouding, or air-fluid levels (which means that air and fluid are seen in the sinuses rather than the expected air alone; Figure 14.1).

In nasal endoscopy, the doctor uses a flexible, fiberoptic instrument to look inside your nose and examine the nasal passages and sinus drainage areas. If infection is present, pus will be seen coming from the openings of the sinuses. Thick sinus tissue resulting from

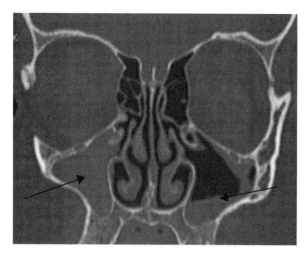

FIGURE 14.1 CT scan of a patient with rhinosinusitis showing the presence of inflammation. Dark black areas are normal sinuses, filled with air; shades of white and gray (*arrow*) indicate the presence of inflammatory tissue in the sinuses, where there should be none.

prior sinus infections is frequently present in individuals who do not have any symptoms. If this is the case, your doctor should examine your nasal structures or get a CT scan before making a diagnosis of rhinosinusitis.

Four Types of Rhinosinusitis

Rhinosinusitis is divided into four categories:

- Acute rhinosinusitis starts suddenly, lasts from 1 day to 4 weeks, and its symptoms usually go away on their own
- Subacute rhinosinusitis lasts from 4 to 12 weeks
- Recurrent acute rhinosinusitis is defined as four or more episodes of acute rhinosinusitis, lasting at least 7 days each, in any 1-year period

- Chronic rhinosinusitis has symptoms that persist for 12 weeks or longer, and acute infectious episodes may be interspersed in this time

Most experts do not believe rhinosinusitis causes headache alone. Sinus headache includes tenderness and pain of the face, nasal congestion, and nasal discharge in the form of pus. It has a deep, dull, aching quality combined with a heaviness and fullness. The pain comes from swollen and inflamed nasal structures. Nausea and vomiting rarely occur. Other signs and symptoms include an inability to smell, pain upon chewing, and bad breath. Upper jaw pain or toothache, poor response to decongestants, and colored nasal discharge can also indicate rhinosinusitis. Migraine and tension-type headaches are often confused with a sinus headache because of similarity in location. However, diagnosing a sinus headache requires clinical, nasal endoscopic, or CT evidence of acute rhinosinusitis and that the headache has developed, worsened, or improved alongside the infection.

Talia, a 21-year-old medical student, reported a new nasal discharge; pain in her face; bad breath; a dull, aching, frontal headache; and a fever of 103°F (39°C). Her temperature returned to normal after several days, but her nasal congestion and postnasal drip did not improve. After the symptoms of her infection were treated, her headache, nasal congestion, and postnasal drip resolved.

Talia had a sinus headache.

Sinus Headache Treatment

The management goals for the treatment of rhinosinusitis are:

- Treat the bacterial infection
- Reduce the swelling in the nasal cavities

- Drain the sinuses
- Maintain open drainage passages

Treating the infection should help treat the headache of rhinosinusitis. Uncomplicated rhinosinusitis is treated with antibiotics for 10 to 14 days. Sphenoid sinusitis, affecting the sinuses in the back of the skull, can be much more dangerous and needs longer, more aggressive treatment.

Steam and saline prevent dried nasal passages and help clear the mucus. Decongestants relieve symptoms by shrinking inflamed and swollen nasal tissues. Nasal spray decongestants should be limited to 3 to 4 days to prevent decongestant rebound (swelling when decongestant use is delayed or stopped). If treatment for more than 3 days is necessary, you should take decongestants by mouth, because oral decongestant medications reduce nasal blood flow without the risk of rebound swelling.

Antihistamines (allergy medications) are not effective in the management of acute rhinosinusitis. Anti-inflammatory topical corticosteroids, creams, or ointments (applied in the nose), available as over-the-counter products or as prescription medications, may be helpful in the treatment of rhinosinusitis.

Confusing Migraine with "Sinus Headache"

Zach, a 34-year-old teacher, was convinced he didn't have migraine. "I don't get migraines; my headaches are sinus headaches." His headaches occurred several times a year. "It must be the weather change," he would remark. Each episode lasted from a day to a couple of weeks, and he had associated nasal congestion. The throbbing headache occurred on the right side of his head, was moderate

(Continued)

(Continued)

in intensity, and was associated with his congestion. "The pain is right here," he said as he pressed his fingers just below the inner corners of his eyes, "I can feel the swelling, and when I press here, it feels better. That's a sinus headache, right?"

Many people with migraine get some kind of sinus pressure during a migraine attack, and therefore may believe—incorrectly—that they have a sinus headache. This mistaken impression exists because tissue may swell within the nose as part of migraine and cluster headaches. Likewise, because weather change can trigger migraine attacks, some people mistakenly think they are having a sinus headache. In fact, changes in weather do not trigger sinus headache. If you have sinus pressure and nasal congestion and do not have a fever, you most likely have a headache of migraine. Many of the drugs used to treat sinus headache may help migraine a little, but these drugs can also cause medication-overuse headache. Unfortunately, the myth of sinus headache has prevented many people from being appropriately diagnosed and treated for their headache of migraine.

If you have rhinosinusitis, you will know it; you will feel sick and have a fever, bad breath, nasal congestion, and colored mucus running from your nose. If you have pain in your sinus area without the symptoms of sinus infection, you most likely have migraine.

Chapter 15

Disorders of the Neck

In this chapter, you'll learn:

- What cervicogenic headache is
- What can cause cervicogenic headache
- How cervicogenic headache is diagnosed and treated

"It doesn't happen every time, but that's the only time it does happen."
"What are you talking about, Alice?"
"My headaches! It's so weird! They only happen when I tilt my head like this . . . "
"Well, don't do it, for God's sake! You'll get a headache!"
"No, no! That's what I was trying to say. It doesn't happen every time I tilt my head. I'd be going crazy! But that's the only time I do get a headache!"
"You're strange, Alice."

—Lewis Carroll, *Alice in Wonderland*

Actually, the fictional Alice in the above conversation is not so strange at all. She probably has what is called **cervicogenic headache**. As the name implies, cervicogenic headache is a headache generated in the neck: moving or holding the neck in certain positions is the only thing, other than the occasional sneeze or cough, that will bring on an attack or spike a cervicogenic headache. The pain starts in the back of the head and may spread forward. Cervicogenic headache may be due to dystonia, an involuntary posture or movement disorder, or it may be a disorder unto itself. Cervicogenic headache is often confused with chronic migraine. Over half of patients with migraine have neck pain preceding or during a migraine attack. However, headache can also originate in the neck. In fact, many people with chronic migraine also have neck pain, caused or worsened by actual disease in the neck (Figure 15.1).

Many parts of the neck are sensitive to pain: the joints between the cervical vertebrae, the periosteum (a layer of tissue covering bones and joints), the ligaments of the cervical spine, the neck muscles, the cervical nerves, and the vertebral arteries and veins of the cervical spine. Neck discomfort, stiffness, or pain may extend into the shoulders, upper arms, and even the forearms and fingers. Headache may be present on awakening or may begin after the person returns home from work, and it may last several hours. The headache and neck pain can become continuous, with a baseline headache even when the person is in an optimal position, and the pain may change in intensity over the day or week. Starting in the neck or the occiput (the back of the head), the pain sweeps forward. Some patients have pain in the temples, others have neck pain referred to the forehead or half of the head, and some have pain on both sides of the head. "Crunching" sounds in the neck (crepitus) may be present.

Born That Way

Headache referred from the neck has many causes. People with this type of headache may be born with joint hypermobility (joints in the spine of the neck that have excessive mobility) or congenital neck joint fusion (joints that have very limited mobility). Abnormalities of the junction between the head and upper cervical spine that are present at birth frequently cause headaches. Occipital or **suboccipital pain** (pain in the back of the head) occurs in about one-fourth of patients with basilar invagination (an abnormality in which the vertebrae of the neck project into the skull), abnormalities of

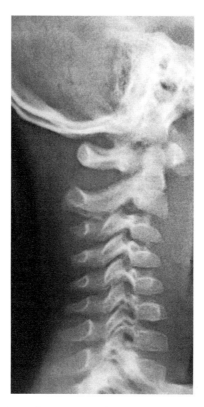

FIGURE 15.1 Cervical spine x-ray showing straightening of the neck due to muscle spasm. Muscle spasms can trigger head pain.

the bones of the head, and Arnold-Chiari malformation, in which part of the brain (the brainstem and the cerebellum) extends into the spinal canal of the neck. The headaches associated with these abnormalities often have features not seen in other headache disorders, such as pain that is felt in the back of the head and triggered by flexing the neck, coughing, or straining. Sometimes the pain has a pronounced postural component, resulting in pain that worsens with standing and is relieved by lying down. Patients may have vertigo (dizziness), facial numbness, weakness of the arms or legs, or ataxia (impaired balance and incoordination) as well as neurologic findings on physical examination. Surgery in patients with these abnormalities often does not relieve the patient's pain.

Got That Way

One can develop problems in the craniovertebral junction (the point at which the skull joins with the spine) and in the upper cervical spine (at the top of the back of the neck), such as tumors, osteomyelitis (bone infection), and multiple myeloma (a form of blood cancer), that produce headache by pressing on the pain-sensitive structures in the upper cervical nerve roots. Blows to the head or forceful sneezing may produce problems with the cervical vertebrae, which can cause persistent occipital headache. Rheumatoid arthritis of the upper cervical spine produces headaches by inflammation of the synovial joints of the neck and by damaging ligaments and nerves of the neck. These disorders produce occipital headaches that are worsened or triggered by neck movements.

Arthritis of the bones of the neck (cervical spondylosis), a common condition for people over the age of 40, may occasionally cause headaches. However, because the arthritis mainly involves the lower part of the neck, cervical arthritis does not usually cause head pain. The restriction of movement in the arthritic lower cervical regions may lead to excessive "play" in the upper neck. Unconsciously, the body tries to maintain its normal movement patterns. To balance the restricted movement of the lower neck, movement of the upper neck may increase. This increased movement is what may produce headache, typically in the back of the head and often on one side.

Trauma

Trauma, such as **whiplash** injuries to the neck in a car accident or neck hyperextension after tracheal tube placement during an operation, can bring on headache (see Chapter 16). Whiplash causes injury to the upper cervical ligaments and muscles, which results in self-limited neck, occipital, and, occasionally, frontal pain that clears within days or a few weeks. Maintaining the same neck position for a long period is common in people who have certain occupations, especially musicians and people who work on a computer.

Dystonia

Dystonia, involuntary muscle spasms that bend and twist the neck, is not a disease but a syndrome characterized by abnormal movements or defective positioning of the affected parts of the body. Focal dystonias occurring in the head and neck region are called **craniocervical dystonia**. Craniocervical dystonia is often encountered in middle-aged adults. The underlying muscular hyperactivity may cause abnormal movements or a fixed defective position. It may cause jerky, repetitive movement or rhythmic movements like a tremor. The pain of dystonia of the neck is due to continuous contraction of muscles or is a result of nerve irritation caused by the muscular hyperactivity.

Diagnosis and Treatment

Cervical spine disorders are believed to be a common cause of headache, because pain often is located in the neck and back of the head, but neck pain is present in most migraine attacks and many tension-type headaches. Therapy always starts with a thorough investigation to identify a cause. Diagnosis of headache caused by a neck disorder requires satisfying specific criteria. The headache must occur in the neck and back of the head, but radiation to other parts of the head or neck is possible. The headache may occur on one or both sides of the head. It must be possible to provoke the pain by means of certain neck movements or positions. The doctor's examination should reveal evidence of restricted neck movement; changes in the structure, contour, or tone of the cervical muscles; or increased sensitivity to pain on pressing (tenderness). An x-ray of the cervical spine often reveals a straightened neck, with loss of the normal curvature due to muscle spasm as well as arthritis. If you find yourself tilting your head to one side or the rotation of your head on your neck is limited—and especially if it is painful—or your ability to move your upper neck forward and backward is decreased, your doctor may order a CT scan or MRI. Plain x-rays of the skull base are rarely helpful.

The usual treatment for cervicogenic headache is physical therapy. Muscle tenderness may be eased or increased by pressing on the tender muscle with your fingers. A hot shower gives temporary relief. Mobilization, manipulation, massage, deep heat, and other physical methods often give comfort. Some patients may find a cervical collar helpful. A firm foam pad under the pillow or a shaped foam pillow is also often helpful. The usual drug treatment consists of nonsteroidal anti-inflammatory drugs (NSAIDs), such as ibuprofen or naproxen. Some patients need antidepressants, sedatives, or muscle relaxants. Occasionally, your doctor may use a local anesthetic block to relieve the pain (trigger point injections) or a block of the greater occipital nerve. Occipital nerve blocks are also used to treat cluster headache and some cases of migraine. Botulinum toxin (Botox®) is used to treat the cervicogenic component of chronic migraine.

Scott, a 56-year-old man who sits in front of a computer for at least half of his working day, reported having a right-sided headache for several years. He awakened most days with pain, but it usually went away after he showered, shaved, and ate breakfast, only to recur when he sat watching television in the evening. The headache sometimes persisted for the whole day, and, on occasion, it awakened him in the early morning hours.

(Continued)

(Continued)

The pain started in his neck and spread over his ear to his forehead. Stretching his neck or massaging it helped, but neck movements in general were limited. If the pain was moderate, two ibuprofen tablets reduced or abolished the symptoms in about 30 minutes.

Scott had no past neck or whiplash injury but had been a boxer in college.

On examination, his neck was tender and he had trouble moving it from side to side. He was treated with moist heat followed by stretching, and he had significant improvement.

Elizabeth, a 30-year-old woman, developed episodic migraine in her teens. By her mid-20s, she developed daily headache that was typical of chronic migraine. She did not have cough headache or signs of compression of the lower part of the brain. Her doctor discovered she had a small Arnold-Chiari malformation, and she had surgery to correct the malformation. Following the surgery, her headaches were much worse, and she was no longer able to work.

An Arnold-Chiari malformation is something that the person is born with. A small Arnold-Chiari malformation should not be treated surgically unless the patient has significant neurologic findings in addition to the headaches.

Cervicogenic headaches may have many causes, from abnormalities present at birth to arthritis and trauma. The good news is that, like other headaches, physical therapy and medications can usually ease the pain of cervicogenic headache.

Chapter 16

Post-Traumatic Headache

In this chapter, you'll learn:

- What post-traumatic headache is and the difference between acute post-traumatic headache and chronic post-traumatic headache
- What causes post-traumatic headache
- How post-traumatic headache may be treated

Jennifer was a bright, beautiful, 22-year-old woman, and the world was at her feet. She had just graduated from college, was newly married, and had started working in a job that she loved. One day when she was on her way back to the office from lunch, a huge windowpane fell from the skyscraper she was passing, hitting her on the head, knocking her to the ground, and rendering her unconscious.

When she woke up, she felt like one giant ache. Cuts and bruises covered her body. Her face was stitched together, and much of her lovely blonde hair had been shaved away. In less than a heartbeat, her life had radically changed. Strong and determined, Jennifer survived and even triumphed. Her hair grew back. Plastic surgeons repaired her face and her scars healed. But Jennifer is troubled by excruciating headaches. She wakes up in the middle of the night feeling as if an iron band is being tightened around her head. Nothing she takes or does lessens her pain at all.

Like other headache disorders, **post-traumatic headache** has both acute and chronic forms. No one questions the existence of **acute post-traumatic headache**, a headache that begins within 1 week of injury, usually within hours or days of a blow to the head or some other jarring motion. Nausea, light and sound sensitivity, and other features of migraine may accompany the headache. Concentration and memory problems are common, and some people might have trouble managing multiple tasks at once. Vertigo or dizziness may also occur. Sleep disturbances and acquired alcohol intolerance are also common.

Although everyone agrees that acute post-traumatic headache is a legitimate disorder, the diagnosis of **chronic post-traumatic headache**, with symptoms that last many months or become permanent, is controversial. Studies in the United States and Europe suggest that the headache is permanent in 20 percent of individuals who see a doctor for post-traumatic headache, and chronic post-traumatic headache is seen in North America, most of Europe, India, Japan, and many other countries with diverse cultures and legal systems. The legitimacy of post-traumatic headache is undermined by unethical lawyers, legal systems that encourage people who have been in accidents to embellish or manufacture symptoms, and doctors who order tests and treatments to increase damage awards, sometimes causing other doctors and patients to think post-traumatic headache is a made-up disorder. Patients are challenged and stigmatized for having post-traumatic headache—except, perhaps, if it is from a sports injury.

To qualify as chronic post-traumatic headache, pain must persist for more than 3 months. Sleep and mood disturbances are common, as are balance, concentration, and memory problems, which may remain persistent. The features of acute and chronic post-traumatic headache usually resemble more commonly occurring headache disorders, such as chronic migraine (see Chapter 6), chronic tension-type headache (see Chapter 11), and, rarely, cluster headache (see Chapter 12).

When a concussion occurs and a patient has the nonheadache symptoms of concussion as well as headaches, the patient has postconcussion syndrome. Patients with postconcussion headache often have associated problems that may be the cause of major disability. Patients with postconcussion symptoms often report that their memory, concentration, and attention spans are very poor. Yet, despite the patients' severe difficulties in real-life situations, formal testing results are usually normal unless very sophisticated tests are performed. Patients may also suffer from insomnia, and the headache pain and cognitive symptoms may be increased by physical and mental activity. Daily post-traumatic headaches, cognitive problems, legal difficulties, and the belief that chronic post-traumatic headache does not exist as a legitimate medical problem result in a significant decrease in the patients' quality of life.

Causes of Post-Traumatic Headache

Because the neck hinges the head relative to the body and because the brain is fixed to the base of the skull, when trauma occurs, most of the linear, forward, and backward motion of the body is converted into rotational or circular movement of the brain (Figure 16.1). The nerve axons (the long, thin, threadlike parts of the nerve cells that transfer nerve impulses) are stretched, causing immediate injury that results in an alteration or loss of consciousness. In more severe cases, the axons are detached.

In less severe cases, the axons remain unbroken but do not function normally for a long period of time. Even minor concussions without loss of consciousness can have a long-lasting effect on brain function. Football players with this kind of concussion do worse academically than those who have never suffered a concussion. In some people, a mild acute concussion triggers an immediate visual migraine aura.

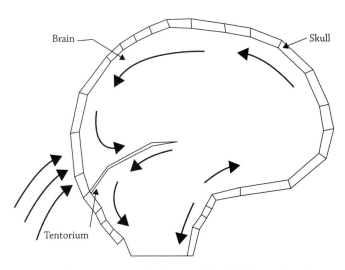

FIGURE 16.1 Movement of the brain in the skull during head injury. Reproduced from Ward C. Status of head injury modeling. Department of Transportation Head and Neck Injury Criteria Consensus Workshop. March 26–27, 1981.

Acute post-traumatic headache may start immediately after injury or within a few days. It is probably due to the stretching of axons and the subsequent release of brain chemicals into the spaces that surround the nerves, altering their function. What is less clear is why the headache and other symptoms resolve in most patients but are permanent in others.

Treatment of Post-Traumatic Headache

No specific treatment exists for post-traumatic headache. Immediately after the injury, physical and mental rest can treat the headache and concussive symptoms. However, prolonged physical and mental rest are thought to be counterproductive. Therefore, post-traumatic headache is treated according to its symptoms. If the headache behaves like migraine, it is treated like migraine, and the same applies to post-traumatic headaches that resemble tension-type headaches or cluster headaches, which are treated like the headache they resemble.

If you had a concussion, you most likely will have neck pain or local tenderness. Your neck pain can be treated with physical therapy. Physical therapists often recommend a home therapy program of stretching exercises you can do every day. Sometimes there may be a **facet joint** injury in the neck, especially with a whiplash injury, and one-sided neck pain radiates to the back of the head. A doctor can anesthetize the injured joint temporarily to relieve the pain. If this works, a procedure called radiofrequency rhizotomy dulls the nerves to the joint for about a year, providing excellent relief. Post-traumatic vertigo may be difficult to treat. Sleep problems may be partially helped with medicine, but a risk is involved in using habit-forming medications. Concentration and memory problems may be addressed by learning strategies that compensate for the problems. Depression may result from a concussion. If it persists, your doctor may recommend medication or cognitive-behavioral therapy.

Chapter 17

Trigeminal Neuralgia

In this chapter, you'll learn:

- What trigeminal neuralgia is
- How trigeminal neuralgia can be treated

Carla was sitting at her desk when suddenly she felt a jolt of severe pain in her lower left jaw that quickly went away. The pain occurred near a tooth on which she had had a crown placed a few months earlier. She made an appointment with her dentist, who tested the tooth by tapping on it with a dental instrument, causing the pain to recur. The dentist concluded that the pain must be coming from the tooth, and he decided a root canal procedure would fix the problem.

Following the root canal, the pain disappeared for a few weeks, but then it returned. This time, the pain attacks began to occur one or two times a day. Carla returned to her dentist, who referred her to an endodontist in case an extra canal needed to be treated. The endodontist repeated the root canal and Carla was again pain-free for a few weeks, after which the pain returned. The endodontist referred her to an ear, nose, and throat (ENT) physician, who concluded Carla had a temporomandibular joint disorder because no abnormality was found on ENT examination. The ENT doctor then referred Carla to an oral surgeon.

(Continued)

(Continued)

Upon examination, the oral surgeon decided that Carla's temporomandibular joints were working normally and then sent her to a neurologist with a diagnosis of possible neuralgia, an intense, typically intermittent pain along the course of a nerve, especially in the head or face. The neurologist examined Carla and agreed that she appeared to have trigeminal neuralgia. The neurologist ordered imaging studies to rule out other causes of Carla's facial pain, and then started Carla on an anti-seizure medication for the pain.

Trigeminal neuralgia, also known as tic douloureux, is a sudden, excruciating burst of pain in the trigeminal nerve, which supplies sensation to the entire face and mouth. The attacks are so severe that patients are often stopped in their tracks. Usually patients have **trigger zones**, distinct areas of the face or mouth that experience an attack of pain when stimulated by even light touch, but not all attacks are provoked by stimulating a trigger zone; many attacks occur spontaneously.

Typically, trigeminal neuralgia causes intense, sharp pains that usually last seconds, but they can last as long as 2 minutes. The attacks are described as lancinating, a term used to describe pain that is severe and stabbing. Many patients equate the pain to an electrical shock.

After each attack, a refractory period occurs, during which another attack cannot be triggered. Trigeminal neuralgia can include periods of remission during which the pain disappears for months or years at a time but then returns.

The cause of trigeminal neuralgia is not fully understood. It is believed to be caused by a loss of the protective outer layer of the trigeminal nerve. This may occur because an artery or vein rubs against the nerve near the nerve's exit from the skull, a condition known as vascular compression. Many of the surgical treatments for trigeminal neuralgia are based on this mechanism and aimed at either guarding the nerve from the blood vessels or at impairing the functioning of the nerve to decrease its activity. Some diseases, such as multiple sclerosis, can cause the loss of the protective covering of the nerve to the face, and a small percentage of patients with these diseases may develop trigeminal neuralgia.

Carbamazepine (Tegretol®), an anticonvulsant medication, was the treatment of choice for trigeminal neuralgia for many years. Oxcarbazepine (Trileptal®) may be safer and has fewer side effects. Gabapentin (Neurontin®) is also effective for many patients. For many patients, medications easily control the pain, while other patients have initial success that dwindles over time, and some patients have only limited success with medications. For the latter two groups, surgical procedures are an option. One common surgical procedure is microvascular decompression, also called the Janetta procedure, in which the offending blood vessel is prevented from constantly pulsating against the nerve, relieving the abnormal pressure on the nerve. An alternative to major surgery, radiosurgery (Gamma Knife), directs radiation precisely to the area where the nerve enters the brain and appears to be effective in relieving the pain of trigeminal neuralgia.

A wide range of **facial pain** syndromes exist, many of which have overlapping features (see also Chapter 18). Diagnosis of trigeminal neuralgia and other facial pain is based on the patient's clinical presentation. No laboratory tests or imaging procedures can confirm the diagnosis. The patient's history is very important in leading the physician to the correct diagnosis. On average, patients who have facial pain will see four to five doctors before being referred to a pain clinic or specialist. Further education of health care providers may lead to more accurate diagnosis and treatment of these disorders.

Chapter 18

Atypical Facial Pain and
Temporomandibular Disorder

In this chapter, you'll learn:

- How atypical facial pain differs from trigeminal neuralgia
- What temporomandibular disorder is
- How atypical facial pain and temporomandibular disorder may be treated with a multidisciplinary approach

Atypical Facial Pain

Joseph, a 40-year-old man, was kicked in the left side of his face by a horse. He lost consciousness and was taken to the local hospital, where he was treated surgically for a fracture of his left orbit, the group of bones that support the left eye.

Joseph made a remarkable recovery and did not lose his eye or his vision. After the surgery, the facial swelling subsided, but the left side of his face was numb and his left eye did not move as well as the right. His surgeons decided to try to repair the nerves and add support to his left eye. Immediately after the surgery, Joseph reported facial pain that radiated into his left upper teeth. The pain would occasionally become more intense for a few days at a time, requiring him to seek seclusion and wait for the pain to subside.

(Continued)

(Continued)

Joseph continued to have facial pain for more than a year after the surgery, as well as a continuous, aching pain in his left upper teeth that got worse when he tried to chew. His teeth were sensitive to mechanical stimulation, such as tapping, grinding, and chewing. He also had numbness in his left, mid-face region, and two to three times a month his pain became much worse for a period of 24 to 36 hours. During these attacks of more severe pain, Joseph suffered from sensitivity to light and the pain became throbbing.

Joseph was evaluated and diagnosed with atypical facial pain due to dysfunction of the sensory nerves in that region. The physical examination showed his teeth to be very sensitive when tapped, but the dental x-rays were normal. His face had a 50 percent loss of sensation to light touch on the left side. He was otherwise healthy and physically appeared normal, except for some slight facial asymmetry from the original trauma.

Joseph was treated with an antidepressant medication for the pain, with excellent pain relief within 1 month. With continued therapy, he could chew without sensitivity, he regained sensation in his face, and the pain became much less severe and less frequent.

The term *atypical facial pain* has been used since 1924 for pain in the facial region that does not fit the criteria for trigeminal neuralgia (see Chapter 17), a chronic pain condition affecting the nerve responsible for sensation in the face. Another term for atypical facial pain is *persistent idiopathic facial pain*, which is useful to represent the part of the facial pain spectrum without obvious nerve damage. Other names are often given to atypical types of facial pain, such as **stomatodynia, atypical odontalgia, phantom tooth pain, myogenic pain, traumatic neuralgia, trigeminal nerve disorder, trigeminal neuropathy, trigeminal neuropathic pain,** and oral and facial dysesthesias. Atypical facial pain, unlike trigeminal neuralgia, is continuous or nearly continuous and has no trigger points.

A variety of inaccurate terms have been used to describe atypical facial pain, and there is a lack of understanding of what causes the pain. This creates problems with patients' acceptance of a diagnosis of atypical facial pain. Basic pain science research is expanding our knowledge of how pain is transmitted by the nervous system, allowing physicians to better understand and treat pain conditions. Pain research, new medication options, and increased clinical interest in the treatment of pain have led to many new ideas and descriptions of the conditions that produce facial pain. This increased scientific activity may result in more specific and accurate diagnoses and more effective treatments of facial pain.

Temporomandibular Disorder

Ashley was a 19-year-old college student who had a history of clicking in her jaw whenever she opened her mouth. The clicking had been present for 2 years, had never been painful, and had never resulted in any problems with chewing or talking. Unfortunately, during a basketball game, Ashley was bumped in the jaw. She woke up the next morning unable to open her jaw. The clicking noises were no longer present, and it was painful to open her mouth more than an inch.

Ashley went to her doctor for an evaluation and was diagnosed as having an anterior displacement of the articular disk in her left temporomandibular joint. In other words, the cartilage disk in her joint had slipped forward and was preventing her from opening her mouth normally. Every time she tried to open her mouth, she was stretching tissues full of blood vessels and nerves, causing the pain. The joint itself was sore from the trauma it had received during her game.

(Continued)

(Continued)

Ashley was treated with anti-inflammatory medications, one week of jaw rest followed by physical therapy, and an oral night guard. Her symptoms eventually subsided, and her jaw was unlocked by the physical therapy exercises. It returned to clicking after 6 weeks.

Ashley's diagnosis was a **temporomandibular disorder**, or **TMD**. TMD is a term that encompasses multiple different diagnoses. Generally, TMDs can be split into two major groups: disorders involving the joint and disorders involving the muscles used for chewing. The joint-related disorders include problems with the disk in the joint, arthritis of the joint, temporomandibular joint trauma, tumors, and congenital malformations of the joint. The muscular disorders include spasm, muscle fatigue, regional muscle pain (**myofascial pain**), infections, and trauma to the muscles. Treatment of TMDs is individualized according to the findings on the patient's evaluation.

TMD involving the muscles is often self-limiting. It can be treated with aspirin, acetaminophen, or ibuprofen; a soft diet; and application of warm compresses. Physical therapy includes opening and closing the jaw and moving it from side to side for 5 minutes at least three times a day for 2 weeks. Medications also used to relieve pain include tricyclic antidepressants and muscle relaxants. Botulinum toxin (Botox®) can be used to treat muscle spasm and pain. The most common dental treatment is use of splints or bite plates for a short period. Splints are clear plastic appliances that fit between the upper and lower teeth. They reduce grinding and clenching (bruxism) and relieve muscle tension and pain. Treatment of joint-related TMD can include many of the above treatments but may also require surgical intervention.

In very difficult cases, a **multidisciplinary approach** is often recommended, meaning that many specialists, including ear, nose, and throat (ENT) physicians; dentists; neurologists; physical therapists; and psychologists or psychiatrists may work together to make a diagnosis. You should question your diagnosis if your treatment is not working.

As stated earlier, patients with facial pain frequently see multiple doctors from many specialties before being given an appropriate diagnosis and a course of treatment that helps their pain. These multiple doctor visits, referrals, and treatments not only are frustrating for the patient who is in pain but also are quite costly. Many physicians treat the face, head, and neck, and, unfortunately, TMD has become a generalized label for a variety of pain syndromes. The good news is that TMD pain syndromes are now better understood through research and are diagnosed more quickly by educated physicians.

GLOSSARY

Abdominal migraine: a migraine equivalent (often not recognized as such) characterized by recurrent attacks of abdominal pain, usually occurring in children

Acute post-traumatic headache: headache that begins within a week of injury, usually within hours or days of a blow to the head or some other jarring motion

Acute treatment: medications that abort a headache, also known as attack treatment

Allergic rhinitis: medical word for hay fever, an allergic reaction that may seem to be a chronic cold. Symptoms include nasal congestion, a runny nose (with clear fluid), sneezing, nose and eye itching, and tearing of the eyes.

Allodynia: sensitivity to touch

Alternating hemiplegia: recurrent episodes of paralysis on one side of the body

Aneurysm: a blood-filled bulge caused by a weakened blood vessel wall

Anxiety: fear or nervousness about what might happen

Atypical odontalgia: also known as atypical facial pain, phantom tooth pain, or neuropathic orofacial pain: is chronic pain in a tooth or teeth, or in a site where teeth have been extracted, or after endodontic treatment, without an identifiable cause

Aura: a sensory perception (warning symptom) that can occur before a migraine and can last through the migraine, although usually it lasts 5 to 60 minutes

Benign: not harmful

Benign paroxysmal vertigo: harmless dizziness that comes and goes suddenly

Biofeedback: "feedback" from a body function that the patient uses to learn to control that body function; found in scientific studies to be highly successful in helping to manage migraine

Botulinum toxin: or Botox®, is an FDA-approved effective treatment for chronic migraine

Brain tumor: a growth of the brain or its covering; a headache caused by a brain tumor can resemble any type of primary headache, but it especially resembles a migraine or tension-type headache

Butterbur: botanical used as a migraine preventive

Cannabis: botanical (marijuana) used as a migraine treatment from 1842 until 1942, but its effectiveness as acute or preventive treatment is unknown

Cervicogenic headache: headache that is generated in the neck

Childhood periodic syndromes: different kinds of migraine that don't usually cause headache. They include cyclic vomiting, abdominal migraine, benign paroxysmal vertigo (dizziness), alternating hemiplegia of childhood (weakness or paralysis), and benign paroxysmal torticollis (spasms of the neck muscles).

Chronic migraine: migraine occurring more than 15 days a month

Chronic post-traumatic headache: headache that continues for more than 3 months after head injury

Chronic tension-type headache: a tension-type headache occurring on 15 days or more every month for 3 months

Cluster headache: one-sided pain centered in or around the eye

Coexistent: illnesses that occur in the migraine patient at a rate that would be expected by chance

Comorbid: conditions existing simultaneously with, and usually independently of, another medical condition. An example is migraine and irritable bowel syndrome (IBS): both IBS and migraine occurring in the same person in the same time period are comorbid.

Computed tomography (CT): an imaging procedure. CT is the best way to evaluate the sinuses because it may show thickening of the surface of the sinuses, scarring, clouding, or air-fluid levels (which means that air and fluid are seen in the sinuses rather than the expected air alone).

Craniocervical dystonia: focal dystonia occurring in the head and neck region

Cyclic vomiting: recurrent, prolonged attacks of severe nausea and vomiting

Depression: a serious medical condition in which a person feels very sad, hopeless, and unimportant

Diastolic blood pressure: blood pressure is a measurement of how open your blood vessels are, and it is expressed as two numbers. The bottom number, your diastolic blood pressure, indicates the pressure when your heart relaxes and prepares for its next pump.

Disability: limitations in one's day-to-day activities or occupation because of an impairment

Dissection: a rupture of the lining of an artery

Dystonia: involuntary muscle spasms that bend and twist the neck

Electrocardiogram: a common test that records the electrical signals in your heart and that is used to detect heart problems and monitor the heart's status

Encephalitis: inflammation of the brain

Epilepsy: a seizure disorder. Migraine and epilepsy are comorbid: if you have one disorder, you are more likely to have the other.

Episodic tension-type headache: dull pain, tightness, or pressure around your forehead or the back of your head and neck that occur less than 15 days per month

Estrogen: the hormone that controls a woman's monthly cycle

Facet joints: small joints located between and behind each vertebra

Facial pain: pain felt in any part of the face, including the mouth and eyes

Feverfew: botanical used as a migraine preventive

Fibromyalgia: chronic widespread pain, tenderness, and stiffness of muscles that is usually accompanied by fatigue, headache, and sleep disturbances

Headache: pain in the head or neck areas

Headache calendar: used for tracking headaches and headache triggers for a few months. Best if used before seeing a headache specialist.

Headache treatment: acute or preventive medicine, lifestyle changes, or mindfulness (biofeedback or yoga) to manage headaches

Hemicrania continua: headache that is continuous but is always on only one side of the head

Hemiplegic migraine: attacks of one-sided weakness with migraine. Often starts in childhood and stops in adulthood. Starts with visual aura of migraine, followed by the onset of slowly progressive, one-sided numbness or pins and needles, and then weakness on that side.

Hypertension: high blood pressure. High blood pressure does not cause headache unless the numbers are very high, which would be a true medical emergency.

Ice pick headache: brief, sudden, and severe jabs of pain that last seconds

International Headache Society (IHS): a group whose pupose is to advance headache science, education, and management and to promote worldwide headache awareness

Intracranial pathology: the presence of injury, bleeding, tumor, or abscess in the head

Lumbar puncture: (also known as a spinal tap) a medical procedure in which a needle is inserted between two lumbar bones (vertebrae) to remove a sample of cerebrospinal fluid

Medication: in headache treatment, medicines are acute (they stop a headache) or preventive (they keep headaches from happening)

Meningitis: an infection of the cerebrospinal fluid and the linings covering the brain. The headache in meningitis is usually felt on both sides of the brain, is generally severe, and worsens relentlessly over hours or days.

MIDAS: Migraine Disability Assessment form used to determine your level of disability due to migraine

Migraine: a medical condition that usually causes a pounding, throbbing headache on one side of the head

Migraine in children: in younger children, attacks are often shorter and occur on both sides of the head. As children get older, they develop one-sided headache. Children frequently experience nausea and/or vomiting with their headaches.

Migraine research: looking to find the causes, better treatment, and a cure for migraine

Migraine with aura: the official name for a headache preceded by a neurologic symptom that changes over 5 to 60 minutes. Most commonly, auras are visual, but they can involve other sensory systems.

Migraine with brainstem aura: aura coming from the back of the brain. Symptoms may be on both sides of the visual fields and can lead to temporary blindness, vertigo, double vision, or lack of coordination.

Migraine without aura: (previously called common migraine) headache that lasts for a defined period of time, usually hours, and is accompanied by sensitivity to light and/or sound or by nausea

Multidisciplinary approach: composed of, or combining, several usually separate branches of medical expertise

Myofascial pain: pressure on sensitive points in your muscles (trigger points) causes pain in unrelated parts of your body

Myogenic pain: muscle pain

Nasal endoscopy: the use of a flexible, fiberoptic instrument to look inside your nose and to examine the nasal passages and sinus drainage areas

New daily persistent headache: a subtype of chronic daily headache in which a persistent headache starts on a single day and continues as constant, relentless pain. It may otherwise resemble chronic migraine or tension-type headache.

Obesity: having too much body fat

Osmophobia: sensitivity to odors

Pain: an unpleasant, mild to agonizing physical sensation

Paroxysmal hemicrania: a very rare, clusterlike headache that mainly affects women. The attacks are one-sided, centered on the eye, excruciatingly severe, and accompanied by tearing, drooping of the eyelid, and facial swelling on the side of the headache. Attacks are shorter than cluster headache attacks but are more frequent.

Paroxysmal torticollis: spasms of the neck muscles

Phantom tooth pain: persistent pain in the area from which a tooth has been extracted

Phonophobia: sensitivity to noise

Photophobia: sensitivity to light

Physical therapy: physical treatments of muscle used to strengthen neck muscles, improve mobility, and correct poor posture, thus treating headache

Postconcussive headache: headache after mild brain injury

Post-traumatic headache: headache after head trauma

Preventive treatment: medications that over weeks or months prevent headaches and do not work on an acute attack

Primary headache: the headache itself is the main medical problem

Progesterone: a female sex hormone that prepares and maintains the uterus for pregnancy

Rebound headache: headache that occurs when headache medications are overused

Relaxation: a stress-management technique for those whose headaches are brought on by stress

Rhinosinusitis: acute sinusitis, an infection of one or more of the cranial sinuses (air-filled cavities in the skull)

Riboflavin: vitamin B_2, used as a migraine preventive

Secondary headache: headache that is a result of an underlying medical condition, such as a neck injury or a sinus infection

Sexual activity headache: most often an explosively sudden and severe headache occurring at or around the time of orgasm. It may also be a warning sign for a subarachnoid hemorrhage from a ruptured cerebral aneurysm; therefore, the first attack of a sexual activity headache is considered a medical emergency and should be seen in the emergency department as soon as possible.

Spinal headache: headache that may be caused by a constant leak of cerebrospinal fluid through a hole in the coverings of the spinal cord. The headache subsides when the person lies down and returns in seconds or minutes when he or she stands. It usually starts in the back of the head or upper neck and spreads over the entire head.

Spinal tap: (also known as a lumbar puncture) a medical procedure in which a needle is inserted between two lumbar bones (vertebrae) to remove a sample of cerebrospinal fluid

Stigma: the perception of a person's being less worthy than friends and colleagues, or a person's being treated unfairly

Stomatodynia: a burning sensation in the mouth with no underlying dental or medical cause

Stroke: a disruption of the normal blood flow to the brain that causes brain tissue to die

Subarachnoid hemorrhage: blood leaking into the space between the two linings that surround the brain

Suboccipital pain: pain below the back of the skull

Suicide headache: the name for cluster headache that was used before effective treatments were available

Temporomandibular disorder (TMD): disorder involving the temporomandibular joint or disorder involving the muscles used for chewing

Tension-type headache: the most common type of headache, characterized by pain in the head, scalp, or neck and sometimes associated with muscle tightness in those areas

Topiramate: an antiepileptic medicine proven to be an effective migraine preventive

Traumatic neuralgia: a sharp, shocking pain that follows the path of a nerve and is due to irritation or damage to the nerve

Trigeminal nerve: supplies sensation to the entire face and mouth

Trigeminal nerve disorder: an atypical type of facial pain

Trigeminal neuralgia: a sudden, excruciating burst of pain in the trigeminal nerve, also called tic douloureux

Trigeminal neuropathic pain: an atypical type of facial pain

Trigeminal neuropathy: damage or pathologic change to the trigeminal nerve

Trigger zones: distinct areas of the face or mouth that experience an attack of pain when stimulated by even light touch

Triptan: specific acute migraine medication

Whiplash: an injury that causes the neck to move either forward to backward or backward to forward with more force than is normal

Tests that May Help Patients with Headache

Laboratory tests are not necessary for diagnosis if you are a typical healthy patient with migraine or someone who is experiencing tension-type headache, but they may be helpful prior to treatment. An electrocardiogram may be needed if risk factors for heart disease are present or as a baseline prior to the use of triptans, ergots, or other vasoconstricting drugs. An erythrocyte sedimentation rate (ESR) (also called simply *sedimentation rate*) measures inflammation in the body and can establish the diagnosis of giant cell arteritis, which is a cause of headache and sudden blindness in the elderly.

Computed tomography (CT) uses a computer to analyze multiple x-rays to produce better images. In contrast, magnetic resonance imaging (MRI) uses a computer, a powerful magnet, and radio waves to analyze the area of the body in question. CT and MRI are not needed if you have migraine, if no recent change in your headache pattern has occurred, you have no history of seizures, and you have a normal neurologic examination.

Magnetic resonance angiography uses MRI to examine arteries. It is a screening tool for suspected aneurysms (weakened areas of blood vessel that pouch outward) or arteriovenous malformations (abnormal tangles of vessels). Magnetic resonance venography looks for evidence of a blood clot or obscuration in the veins or venous sinuses (very different from sinuses of the nose) that drain blood from the brain.

A **lumbar puncture**, also called a spinal tap, involves placing a needle through the space between two vertebrae in the low back into a pocket that contains the cerebrospinal fluid (CSF). The examiner can measure the CSF pressure and determine whether infection or inflammation is present. A lumbar puncture may still need to be done even if the CT or MRI is normal, because these tests may miss the presence of blood or infection and cannot diagnose increased CSF pressure.

Resources for Patients
with Headache Disorders

American Headache and Migraine Association (AHMA)
19 Mantua Road
Mount Royal, NJ 08061
Tel: 856-423-0043
Fax: 856-423-0082
Email: ahma@talley.com
ahma.memberclicks.net

AHMA is a nonprofit patient–health professional partnership dedicated to advancing the treatment and management of headache and to raising the public awareness of headache as a valid, biologically based illness. Its goals are to empower headache patients through education and to support them by educating their families, employers, and the public in general.

AHMA was created in 2013 through an initiative of the American Headache Society (see below). Its website has extensive resource information, a list of support groups, and much more.

American Headache Society (AHS)
19 Mantua Road
Mt. Royal, NJ 08061
Tel: 856-423-0043

Fax: 856-423-0082

Email: ahshq@talley.com

americanheadachesociety.org

The AHS is an organization of more than 2,400 physicians, health professionals, and research scientists. Its website contains information primarily of interest to clinical professionals. AHS produces educational programs and materials, coordinate its support groups, and undertake public awareness initiatives.

National Headache Foundation

820 N. Orleans

Suite 201

Chicago, IL 60610-3132

Tel: 312-279-2650

Email: info@headaches.org

headaches.org

The Foundation's goals are to serve as an information resource to headache patients, their families, and the health care providers who treat them; to raise public awareness that headaches are a legitimate biological disease and patients should receive understanding and continuity of care; and to promote research into potential headache causes and treatments.

The Foundation's website offers information on a variety of topics related to headache, information on support groups, information about clinical trials, publications, and much more.

Neurology Now® Magazine

333 Seventh Avenue, 19th Floor

New York, NY 10001

NeurologyNow.com

Neurology Now is the American Academy of Neurology's award-winning magazine for patients and caregivers and a trusted resource for anyone interested in brain health. Published six times a year, *Neurology Now* features compelling articles about people living with neurologic disorders, reliable information about the diagnosis and treatment of neurologic diseases, advice on wellness and disease prevention, strategies for coping effectively with neurologic disorders, and more. Print subscriptions are free to individuals with a neurologic disorder, their caregivers, and family members and friends residing in the United States.

National Institute of Neurological Diseases and Stroke (NINDS)
National Institutes of Health Neurological Institute
P.O. Box 5801
Bethesda, MD 20824
ninds.nih.gov

This site contains information of interest to people with a wide range of neurologic disorders, including migraine and other headaches.

About the American Academy of Neurology

The American Academy of Neurology represents 32,000 neurologists and neuroscience professionals and is dedicated to promoting the highest quality patient-centered neurologic care. A neurologist is a doctor with specialized training in diagnosing, treating, and managing disorders of the brain and nervous system such as Alzheimer's disease, stroke, migraine, multiple sclerosis, concussion, Parkinson's disease, and epilepsy.

For more information about the American Academy of Neurology, visit *AAN.com.*

To sign up for a free subscription to *Neurology Now®*, the Academy's magazine for patients and caregivers, visit *NeurologyNow.com.*

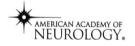

INDEX

Tables, figures, and boxes are indicated by an italic *t*, *f*, or *b* following the page number.